mirror image

w. d. janaway

ISBN: 978-1-9995240-0-5

Front cover image: D-Keine/E+/Getty Images
Back cover and flap image: amtitus/Getty Images

FIN 01 02 2019

FOR YOU

"Sometimes you can't see yourself clearly until you see yourself through the eyes of others."

-- Ellen DeGeneres

mirror
image

1

My younger sister Steffanni is getting married in five months, and I am going to be her maid of honour. Standing atop a two foot square fitting pedestal at the back of Lindman's Bridal Boutique, I studied the woman in the mirror looking back at me. *Was this really me?* Until this very moment, I had never paid too much attention to my appearance or my weight. For that matter, I can't really think of anyone else in my family who has either. Vanity was one of those potentially destructive traits which were thankfully bypassed by all of us. Five minutes ago however, for me all that changed.

As I looked around the fitting area I could see my sister-in-law, Melinda, who is married to my older brother Phillip, relaxing on a viewing sofa. Melinda is a short five feet tall, and she is nine months pregnant, ready to give birth to their first child any day now. Beside her, my mother, Victoria, stood a few feet behind me on another fitting pedestal. I could see her eyes beaming with pride as two sales ladies' trying to communicate with straight pins pinched between their teeth, hemmed a full length, royal blue dress around her ankles. Moments ago however, one of the two sales ladies now helping my mom, was fastening the buttons up the back of my dress. While doing so, and making small talk, she asked me if we knew whether Melinda was having a boy or a girl, and what names if any, she had picked out. Then the sales lady looked straight faced, directly at me, and asked me when my baby was due. Can you believe it? Me? Five foot, two inches tall, one hundred and twenty something pounds, and beyond some unexplainable miracle, definitely not pregnant! Suddenly, obviously rattled and embarrassed by her mistake, the lady rapidly turned and began assisting with mom, deliberately avoiding me at every glance.

Standing before the full wall mirror, I stared curiously; still trying to see what it was that would cause the sales lady to make such a remark. *I'm not fat!* I whispered to myself while sucking in my stomach. I stood up as tall as I could. I straightened my posture, pulled my shoulders back, and my chin up. *Well?* I hesitated. *I'm not that fat,* I thought, shaking my head. Uncertainty however, was slowly creeping in.

"Well?" Steffanni's voice cut into my thoughts, "What do you think of the dress? Do you like it? Don't you just love this material?" She asked, pinching and sliding the hem of my dress through her fingers.

I slowly turned my body from side to side while still looking into the mirror, trying to observe my reflection from every angle.

"Steffi, do you think I am too fat?" I asked her undecidedly.

"Oh please! You Jenni, fat?" She grimaced. "Maybe if you looked like Melinda over there, and were without child."

"What?" I exclaimed sharply, covering my stomach with both hands. "So you do think I am fat and look pregnant too?"

"Hey sis, calm down. That isn't what I said and you know it. Why are you acting so ridiculous all of a sudden? You know you're not fat. You have never been overweight a day in your life," she said pulling my hands down to my sides. "I think the dress looks great, and you look beautiful in it." She paused a moment, a hint of concern changing her smile. "Wait, it's the dress making you crazy isn't it? You don't actually like the dress at all do you? Be honest with me. Do you hate it or don't you?"

I looked away from the mirror to Steffanni, her smile now completely replaced with a worried frown.

"Oh my gosh Steffi no," I reassured her. I stepped down from the pedestal and embraced her in a tight hug. "Honestly sis, I love the dress. It's beautiful. I just think that...." I stopped mid sentence and turned back to the mirror.

"What? You think what Jenni?"

"I just think that maybe it looks better without me in it."

"Oh nonsense," mom joined in our conversation. "It is going to be a beautiful wedding, and both my girls are going to be absolutely stunning in both their dresses." She beamed. "Speaking of which," she said, putting her hands on Steffanni's shoulders turning her back toward the dressing room, "it's time for the rest of us to sit down, and the bride to pick out her gown."

Two hours later, after watching Steffanni try on over a dozen different gowns; the decision was finally narrowed down to two. The toss up was between a regal white chiffon ballroom style gown, and a form fitting open back, Victorian satin, streamline lace gown. Both dresses would have to be custom fit, and would require at least eight weeks to bead the way Steffanni wanted; not including the time needed to design and construct matching headpieces. A decision couldn't wait much longer.

"Your dad would know which dress to go with," said Melinda.

"Oh I agree," mom nodded. "Stuart has always had exceptional insight with things like this. He would be the perfect deciding vote."

Because the boutique had another fitting coming in, we took pictures of Steffanni in each gown, and then made copies of each for her to take with her. Stopping by my parent's house later that night, I found my dad sitting at his desk in his den, looking down at the different photographs. Mom and Steffanni stood at either side of him, pointing out what it was they both liked and disliked with each gown.

"Now if we could just find a good man for your sister," I heard my father chuckling. "You and your sister could have that double wedding the two of you were always parading about. I could purchase both gowns and you could each wear one."

"Oh .Daddy," I blurted while entering the room. "You know you're the only man for me. Besides, I don't think there is a man out there strong enough to carry this body over a thresh-hold."

All three of them glanced up acknowledging my arrival, and then all three of them laughed. Neither of them disputed my 'being too heavy remark', which obviously was not quite the response I needed, or wanted to hear. I waited the rest of the evening, fishing and hoping for any one of them to say I wasn't too fat or overweight but it never happened. The only focus was on the decision at hand as to which dress my sister was going choose. It was as if my being fat enough to be mistaken for a pregnant lady wasn't in any way an issue, just an already known, already accepted everyday fact. When it was eventually decided that the Victorian satin gown was the one that Steffanni would wear, dad teased jokingly that of course we would all have to agree on the more expensive of the two gowns, but in fact he too also preferred it over the other. Steffanni thought it looked nicer in the photo than the other gown did, and therefore would make for a nicer wedding album. When Mom said that she thought the streamline lace in the Victorian satin gown captured Steffanni's slim figure better, Steffanni beamed with delight. I think she made her decision right there and then; and so it was settled. My baby sister was going to be a model bride, and I was going to be her FAT sidekick.

On my way home from my parents house, I made a pit stop at the mall and bought myself a brand new, top of the line digital scale. The only way I was going to know conclusively how overweight I had actually become was to weigh myself. When back at my apartment, I placed my new scale in the far corner of my en-suite bathroom, and apprehensively stepped on. The numbers swiftly flashed up to one hundred and thirty without stopping, and in horror I quickly jumped back. Something must have been wrong. I have never weighed more than one hundred and twenty pounds throughout my entire life! I kicked off my shoes and hesitantly stepped onto the scale again. This time I remained still, and waited until the flashing digits came to a complete stop before I stepped off. The bright red numbers in front of me now displayed a clear one hundred and twenty nine point five pounds. I was shocked. I couldn't believe that number was right, and I spent the next fifteen minutes repeatedly challenging the scale. Every time the red lights went out, I stepped back on and then off again, over and over waiting for the joke to be over, but the numbers didn't sway. Even after I completely undressed, believing surely to have shed a few pounds of clothing, now completely naked, the scale still weighed me in at a clear one hundred and twenty nine pounds. So that was it. I had no choice left but to surrender to the scale, and to accept the truth staring me in the face. The sales lady at Lindman's Boutique earlier that afternoon had been right. I was FAT! I DID look pregnant! It was unquestionably time for me to go on a diet.

2

The following morning I decided to get in some additional early exercise and walk to work instead of driving. I always loved this time of year. It was the second week in April, and although the temperature was still cold enough outside to see your breath as a puff of smoke in the air, the winter's winds had ceased for the season. Signs of the coming spring had begun to unveil themselves from under the light dusting of snow still spread over the ground, and the sun, now rising earlier from its eastern bed, lit up my new found path to work with a warm golden beam. As I walked along, I felt like Dorothy in the Wizard of Oz skipping down the yellow brick road on my way to discovering a whole new world. A world where I myself would not find a heart, or a brain, or courage; but be granted my wish to be thin.

As I approached the Rock Garden Café where I worked, Cindy was standing outside finishing her usual morning coffee and cigarette. I hated seeing Cindy smoking, sabotaging her body her like that. She was only eighteen, and she was a really good kid. When Cindy started working with us a little over month ago I had some reservations about hiring another teenager, but she quickly proved herself more than worthy. She worked hard when she was at the Café, and she always maintained a good-natured manner with customers. Even when dealing with the most difficult of customers, she always maintained her smiling composure. My previous experience working with teenagers here at the Café had proven nothing more than a disappointment when it came to duty and dependability, but Cindy was definitely different. She was soft spoken, almost to a fault at times, and always a pleasure to be around. Because of her maturity and high spirit, customers too are always shocked to find out that she is only eighteen.

On this particular morning however, I noticed something about Cindy that I had not been consciously aware of until now. Her figure. Cindy is a couple of inches taller than I am, maybe about five foot three or four, and I bet she couldn't be more than one hundred and ten pounds soaking wet. Her apron fits smoothly over her abdomen, and she has to keep the straps wrapped twice around her waist just to keep them out of her way so to not trip over them when moving.

"Morning Jenniffer," her sweet voice chirped as I arrived. "Ready for the Saturday rush?"

Saturday mornings at the Café were known to be the busiest shifts. Before noon, I would serve on the average over one hundred cups of coffee and five crates of eggs. Cindy herself would do the same.

"There's a note for you on the counter from Marianne. It says Janice is coming in at ten this morning."

"I didn't have her scheduled for today."

"Yeah, well Marianne apparently told her she could come in. Her note says Janice wanted the extra hours and that she thought with the nicer weather now, we could use her help."

"Help or hindrance?" I sighed. "Maybe I can send her into the kitchen and keep her occupied in there with dishes and things."

"Nice thought, but I doubt it. Marianne asked Toby to come in from seven to three today also. You can read it all in the note for yourself, but Toby's already in the kitchen prepping, and I doubt he will want Janice back there helping him any more than we do out front."

"Great," I sighed. "We are just going to have to do the best we can around her and hope for the best. I'll give her the small group of tables in the far corner, but remember to keep your eyes open, and get to all your new tables as fast as you can."

"Couldn't you just call her around nine or something and tell her that we won't need her help today after all?"

"If I could do that and get away with it without causing a huge fiasco Cindy, you know I would. Trust me. You know as well as I do though, that if Janice asked Marianne for the hours directly, it will be less trouble in the end to just work around her and get the day over with."

"True."

Now don't get the wrong impression here. Janice is a very nice lady, and all of us here at the Café do our best to get along with her. She just isn't a very adept or efficient worker when it comes to waitressing. To put it politely, she's slow, easily confused, and very forgetful. She is friendly enough with the customers, but she is a chatterbox, and a chronic complainer. She just doesn't seem to comprehend that people don't want to sit and listen to all of her stories for five minutes every time their waitress walks by their table letting their meals get cold. Other than the fact that she doesn't have initiative for much more than socializing and complaining about her pay check each week, she absolutely hates the fact that I am her supervisor. She doesn't think it is fair that she should have to listen or answer to someone who is so much younger than herself. Whenever she has a problem or wants something, she runs to Marianne. It doesn't usually bother me too much, but it certainly can be very annoying and frustrating at times. Especially when she gains extra shifts which changes things after I have posted the schedules. Janice is married with three grown children, and her pay check is nothing more than disposable household income which is all allotted for her own extra curricular activities. She herself refers to it as her 'entertainment fund'. Cindy however is working to save for college next fall, and as for me, I'm working to pay rent and trying to build a small nest egg. What for, I am not yet sure, but at least someday when I decide what that is, the finances will be there. Cindy and I need our tips, and we work hard and fast to get them. Janice knows this, which makes it even all the more aggravating when she goes over my head for shifts from Marianne. Honestly, if I could just let Janice go, I would have done so a long time ago. Not just because she undermines my authority either, but strictly because of her work performance. She is Marianne's good friend however, so I imagine she will be at the Café as long as she wants, or her and Marianne's friendship lasts. That is how she got the job here last summer to begin with. One day she and Marianne came in for brunch, and she made a comment about how she would love to work at a nice little place like this to pick up a few extra spending dollars. Before I knew it, she was working here. I didn't even see a resume or be consulted, and I have been managing the Café for ten years now. It's not the career I originally set my goals for, but I do enjoy it, and it does pay the bills. Like Cindy, I started working here straight out of highschool to finance college but for one reason or another, in spite of everything, I never made it out of this small town of Edson, and remained at the Café. After I'd been here a couple of years, the Walkers, Ken and Marianne, went on a six month trip to England and left me in charge. When they returned, I received a very generous bonus for running the place in their absence, and was offered a promotion to management with a substantial salary. It was a very good offer at the time which I would have been crazy to pass up so I graciously accepted. The Rock Garden Café is a third generation business for the Walkers, but they have no children of their own, and want to sell within the next ten years and move back to England. Ken always says they think of me like the daughter they never had, and has made it quite clear they would like for me to buy them out when they decide to sell. They say that at least then, in a sense, a part of them would feel as if the Café remained within their family circle. My family says I'm twenty eight now and it's time to forget any of my previous dreams of going to college and settle down. In their opinion they think I am too old now, and I am at present in 'a good place'. "You are set for life with that offer," Dad always says. "You should take it." In all reality, I know the Café would be a good investment for a single person like myself, and when the Walkers are ready to sell in a few years my nest egg should have enough in it to buy the Café from them outright. Then I would be a business owner with a nice property, and not a glorified waitress or manager anymore, but I still question if that is what I really want. I really don't know what I will do when and if the opportunity arises, but if the last ten years are a precursor, I imagine that I will most likely just buy the Café as expected, and remain here in Edson like everyone else.

"Shall we?" Cindy motioned toward the front doors, butting out her cigarette, while looking at her watch. "Mr. Kingsbury will be here in five."

Mr. Kingsbury was always our first customer each Saturday morning, seven a.m. sharp. He is always the same, a dark roast decaf, a garden breakfast special over easy with rye, and he has never missed a Saturday morning I can remember in twelve years. He is also a generous ten dollar tip that Cindy and I always share. After that, it is each wait staff to their own. Unlike some employers, I never asked or made it mandatory that any of the staff have to share gratuities. I believe that if they work hard enough to earn a tip, then they should get to keep it. Fair as fair.

As the day went on, the hours for me seemed to pass more quickly than usual. Partially due to an additional steady flow of customers streaming in, and partially due to my ulterior new interest with food. I was completely preoccupied by customers' appearances and all the foods they were ordering. For the first time ever, I was consciously aware that men and women did in fact exhibit quite different eating habits. I wondered if Cindy had ever made the same association without looking for it, and caught her attention while she was blending a strawberry milkshake.

"Have you ever noticed that women always seem to take longer to decide on what to order than men do?" I asked her quietly.

"Yeah, of course. Why? You never noticed that before?"

"No. Why do you think that is?"

"Most likely because they are counting menu calories, and calculating plate worth I suppose."

"They are doing what?" I asked, now really confused. "What on earth is plate worth?"

"The total calories served on each plate. You know, what each plate is worth in calories. Like gold."

I passed her a straw.

"You mean you have been working in this industry for over ten years and this is the first time you have ever heard the term plate worth?" She asked me seemingly astonished.

I nodded my head yes without speaking, feeling somewhat naive.

"Unbelievable," she said before walking away. "I thought for sure you would have been able to quote off the top of your head, every food value and plate worth in this entire place on cue."

At the end of our shift later that day, without trying to come across even more simple-minded, I couldn't help but carry on the conversation further with Cindy on our way out.

"Hey Cindy, regarding what we were talking about earlier, is that how you keep your slim figure, by counting these calories and figuring out the plate worth of your meals before you eat?"

"Sometimes." She stated matter of fact. "I don't always calculate everything though. You know I like my chocolate cookies way too much to let their number stop me from eating them. Then there are the French fries here of course?"

"Of course, and we both know you can't have those without Ken's homemade gravy, right?" I answered smiling, while inside wondering exactly what their plate number would be worth.

"Yeah, that's right," she said laughing, waving her hand. "Well I have to go, but I'll see you Monday Jenni. Enjoy your day off."

"You too." I waved back, heading in the opposite direction.

Instead of rushing directly home, I again walked the garden path, this time continuing it behind the Café and all then all the way along the river into town, and went into the bookstore. Quickly I found and opened a copy of Webster's New World Dictionary, and flipped through the pages; my mind reeling with excitement in hopes of unlocking this secret code of silence in the world of being thin. And then there it was in bold black print.

"CALORIE: A UNIT USED FOR MEASURING THE ENERGY PRODUCED BY FOOD WHEN OXIDIZED IN THE BODY"

So that was it. I had found it. The Holy Grail was a calorie. All I had to do to be thin was count and keep track of the calories I ate at each sitting, or my plate worth as it was called compared to the calories I expended throughout my daily routines. I smiled feeling quite proud at my new discovery. It all sounded simple enough. The secret wasn't hidden in whether you ate chocolate cake or not, but how many chocolate cake calories you ate. Now knowing the secret, excitedly I went directly over to the health and beauty section of the store. Surprisingly, there were more than a dozen different books on the subject of calories alone. An hour later, after briefing each one, I finally decided on four. The Calorie Counter's Bible, Every Woman's Guide To Counting Calories, the All In One Dieter's Resource Guide which included a five page list of calories burned during different activities, and lastly, a copy of the Counting Calories For The Woman On The Go pocketbook. That one was even small enough to carry in my purse wherever I went, and included over twenty pages of different franchise fast food listings.

One hundred and sixteen dollars later, and I was home. I collected some paper and pencils, sat down at my kitchen table and spread my new books out in front of me. Looking around, the one conclusion I had made so far was that dieting indeed was definitely not cheap. The rest of my night however, I sat making lists of everything on the menu at The Rock Garden Café, and calculating their corresponding plate worth. To be absolutely sure I was correct in my calculations with all the homemade items such as Marianne's chocolate fudge cookies, I first wrote down lists of the compiled ingredients, and then divided them by the total number of units produced by each recipe.

Until now, every day I ate two of Marianne's homemade peanut butter chocolate chunk cookies at my first break, and two of her chocolate fudge macadamia nut cookies with my coffee at my second break. According to my new calculations, I quickly learned that I consumed nine hundred and twenty four calories every shift I worked in those four cookies alone. *No wonder I looked pregnant!* According to my further findings, one pound was apparently equated to three thousand, five hundred calories, and that meant that I had already eaten more than a quarter of a pound of excess calories so far today, and that included all the additional negative calories I burned by walking to and from work. With that realization, my first dieting resolution was made. *I love chocolate. I love peanut butter. I am never eating either one of them again.*

3

I woke up the following morning feeling tired from my late night of research, but still I was very motivated. I decided to set my goal weight at one hundred and eight pounds. I figured that if I could look as good in the dress I had to wear at Steffanni's wedding as Cindy did in her apron at work, the photographer wouldn't need a wide angle lens just to fit me into the pictures. I was determined not to embarrass my sister by looking like a cow stuffed into a green dress at her ceremony, or in her wedding pictures. At one hundred and eight pounds I thought, everything would look and be okay.

If I were seriously going to be in shape for the wedding in time, this meant I had to lose about one pound each week from now until then, so I decided to start keeping track of my caloric input and output on a daily basis. This seemed to be the only possible way I was sure to stay on track, and be ready for the wedding in time. It didn't take me long however, before I realized that my system wasn't as foolproof as I had originally thought. At the end of the first week, my log book showed that I had burned off about four thousand, seven hundred more calories than I had consumed, yet my scale showed I still weighed the same. I didn't understand, but even more so, I was angry! If all my new books were correct, and three thousand, five hundred calories was equivalent to one pound, I should have lost an entire pound plus a little more and therefore been ahead of schedule. According to my new scale though, I still weighed in at one hundred and twenty nine pounds. It didn't make any sense to me at all. How could a person that committed so much time and energy, vigilance, and dedication to dieting and weight loss, not lose any weight at all? It was no wonder I thought, that people get so depressed when dieting. Worst of all though, I was now an entire week behind in my schedule! Angrily I flipped open my logbook to the next blank page, and wrote in large bold capital letters, **NEW RULES: ONE POUND NOW EQUALS SEVEN THOUSAND NEGATIVE CALORIES, AND ALL CALORIES BURNED, ARE DIVISIBLE BY TWO!** Then I wrote underneath, **ALWAYS ROUND UP FOR INTAKE, AND DOWN FOR OUTPUT!!** Surely these new rules would have to work for me now.

Next, I removed and dumped out my candy dish that always sat in the centre of my living room table, and I replaced it with my logbook. Then I went to work cleaning out my kitchen. I spent six hours reading the back of every boxed and canned food item I owned, and cross referenced each ones' nutritional information with all four of my new books. Any item I found that I thought was too fattening or didn't have its nutritional value labelled well enough for my calculations, I put into a large cardboard box in the front hallway. After emptying all my cupboards and my refrigerator, I then rearranged the remaining contents in a safe and specific order. I designated the refrigerator space for the dairy food group and perishable products, and placed them with the lowest calorie content front to back, top shelf to bottom shelf.

I designated my cupboards each also by different food groups or category, and again put back all the items I kept in the same lowest to highest caloric order front to back. My largest cupboard I assigned for my free foods, which were the ones I could consume as much of as I wanted to at any time, like plain popcorn, broth soups, black coffees, and herbal teas. When I was finished, I proudly dragged the overflowing box containing the *'too fattening for consumption foods'* from the hallway to my car, and drove downtown where I donated all of them to the local Food Bank. I went to my Financial Bank next where I withdrew two thousand dollars form my 'nest egg' savings account, and drove to the mall where I purchased a brand new treadmill. It wasn't just any treadmill either. I needed the best of the best to be sure I wouldn't make any more calculating mistakes. The one I chose not only would track my calories burned during its use, but also my time, distance, speed, incline level, and also monitor my heart rate and blood pressure when activated, all at the touch of a button. I had it delivered later that evening, and devised a strict exercise routine that coincided with my work schedule. I also designed a new goal weight success chart, and tacked it up on my bathroom wall above my scale. My surroundings were shaping up, and now I had to start with me.

For the next three weeks, things went pretty smoothly. Melinda gave birth to a healthy, very cheerful baby girl, and I became the Aunt to Theresa Lyndsay Klark, eight pounds, six and a half ounces. As a new Dad, my brother Phillip beamed with pride. Anyone that saw him looking at his daughter could easily see that he was going to be a great father. The pride and joy he felt inside lit up his eyes like the sparkle on a Christmas tree. I knew that if Phillip was half as good the father to my newborn niece he was as my big brother, little Theresa would be the luckiest girl ever born in Edson.

As for my new found diet, it had finally started working for me, and it was moderately showing some results. A few of my clothes seemed to fit more loosely, and my scale encouraged a beginning nine and a half pound loss. At work, Marianne had noticed the demand for her homemade cookies dropping by nearly two dozen a week, and Cindy continually rolled her eyes, frowning at my deliberate new restrictions. During our break yesterday morning, she even gave me a scolding look and shook her head as she watched me stir two level tablespoons of milk into my coffee. Since the first time I had tasted the bitter beverage years ago, I had always taken my coffee double, double. When a customer introduced me to the calorie reducing benefits of artificial sweetener a couple of weeks back though, I stopped using sugar altogether. I now took my coffee with two thirds of an ounce of milk, not cream, and one sweetener packet. I don't know if I will ever get used to the taste of aspartame, but to me it was worth the sacrifice. I had reduced my coffee by forty five calories per cup which equalled to approximately one hundred and thirty five calories per day, nine hundred and forty five calories per week, or an entire pound of additional fat per month I had until now been consuming. Soon I would develop a new taste for the purity of the bean itself, and start to drink my coffee black.

"Jenni," Cindy questioned curiously watching me. "Are you going to drink that coffee or turn it into a science experiment?"

I didn't answer and turned away. Then she started in with her reprimanding lecture.

"You're really taking this diet and calorie thing to heart, but don't you think you might be overdoing it a little? I mean, you seem to be getting really carried away with it. If you're not careful you know, before you realize it, the calories and this new diet of yours will be controlling you."

"Nothing controls me but me Cindy, and if a simple little diet could control a person, then we wouldn't have an obesity problem in the world today, now would we?"

"All I am saying is just to be careful. Okay Jenni."

"Careful with what? All I am doing is applying some of the new weight control practices I am learning. Things may I remind you, that you thought I already knew."

"True enough, but, well.... look, maybe it's none of my business, and deny what you want, but I can see what you are doing, even though you can't."

This was the first time since I'd met Cindy that she ever remotely started to annoy me in any way.

"Okay." I demanded defensively, "Since you know so much more than me, enlighten me then. Just what exactly is it that I am supposedly doing I need to be careful about?"

"Give it up already will you Jenni. You know exactly what I am talking about. You have cut out all of your favourite foods from your diet. You never eat lunch anymore, and whenever you do eat or drink anything, it is usually something you don't even like! Just how much weight are you going to force your body to lose, before you start feeding it again?"

"What are you talking about? I eat all the time!" I snapped back at her. "And I've hardly lost any weight at all!"

"Oh really? Well whatever you say then boss. But anyone who looks at you can plainly see that you have."

I gulped the rest of my coffee and stood up to get back to work. When I turned, Cindy reached out and firmly grabbed my wrist.

"Look Jenni, all I'm suggesting is for you to be careful okay. I knew this girl last year who started a diet the very same as you have. Before too long, just like you the numbers controlled her too. She landed her skinny little butt in the hospital during the middle of senior year and I never saw her again."

I jerked my wrist back from her grasp, now intentionally rolling my eyes at her.

"That is just craziness Cindy, and I'm not crazy. For heaven's sake, I am simply just trying to get in better shape for my little sister's wedding by shedding a few extra unwanted pounds. I don't see anything wrong with that. You however, are acting like it's some kind of crime or something."

"I may have only known you for a few months now, but I do care about you Jenni, and I just don't want to see you overdo it okay. Besides, if you ended up sick and had to take time off work, I'd be stuck here working with Janice covering all your shifts every day, and she'd be my boss!"

I wanted so much to be angry with Cindy for budding so far into my personal life where she had no business, but I couldn't be. Entertained by the sudden thought of her and Janice working together every day, and the pleading look in her eyes caused me to chuckle out loud knowingly. I reassured her that she was worrying for nothing, and that I was well aware of what I was doing, and my boundaries. And indeed I was. Maybe not necessarily in the way she wanted, but in the only way I could now make things work for me.

At home that night before changing out of my work uniform, I stood sideways in front of my full length closet mirror, and studied my figure. Could Cindy really tell that I had lost some weight? Could others I wondered? I untied my apron and pulled the strings as tightly around my waist as I could. Cindy may be able to see that I had lost weight. My scale may confirm that I had lost weight. The mirror in my bedroom however, still reflected an image to me that didn't really look any thinner at all.

4

With only fifteen weeks left to get in shape for Steffanni's wedding, losing weight for me was becoming harder and harder. In order to keep losing, I had to keep decreasing my caloric intake whilst increasing my exercise. I ran five miles before work, did an hour of aerobics after work, and walked an hour and a half on my treadmill before bed. I can't remember when or even why for that matter, but somewhere along the way I had started counting by two's while I worked out, and somehow I had become stuck on the number fourteen. With every step I took, every knee bend, every stomach crunch, and even every bite I chewed, I counted in a repeating rhythm. *Two-four-six-eight-ten-twelve-four-teen, two-four-six-eight-ten-twelve-four-teen.* I had become a human calculator.

Now weighing in at my original set goal weight of one hundred and eight pounds, I had an additional four pounds still to go to reach my new goal weight of one hundred and four. I expended every calorie I could, and couldn't comfortably allow myself to ingest any more than five hundred calories per day. I loaded my stomach with cups of black coffee, green tea, and bottles of water to chase away any hunger. Most of the time, I could go three to four days without any awareness of a single hunger pang, but then inversely I had days when the more I denied myself food, the more I craved it. Sometimes I just wanted to eat, and for no other reason than to eat. More disturbing too, was the fact that what I wanted to eat was anything and everything. It didn't matter what it was, and in the heat of that moment I didn't care. If it was something in the food category I wanted to eat it, and I wanted to eat all of it. Those moments I was tempted to break my rules and give in to the nagging hunger were the worst. I had come so far, and I knew if I even allowed myself that one extra calorie now, it could be fatal to my breakthrough.

Constipated, bloated, and in pain to the point where any exercising or walking on my treadmill tonight was an incapability, I knew I had to find some new fulfilment. Exhausted and feeling horribly defeated, I sat on my sofa balancing a huge bowl of un-buttered popcorn on top of my very fat, still pregnant looking stomach. I counted each fluffy kernel in my fourteen count rhythm as I popped each kernel in my mouth, and then chewed it slowly fourteen times before swallowing. For a moment, I entertained the thought that maybe Cindy had been right in her worries a few weeks ago about the numbers taking over, and that maybe my dieting formalities possibly had gotten out of hand. Then, just as quickly I dismissed the thought. In order to reach my goal and be thin in time for Steffi's wedding, I had to keep track of everything. I didn't have any other choice. If I didn't remain focussed on the numbers, undeniably I would lose track and fail. It was simple logic, and therefore I knew I was still in complete control.

I clicked on my television and flipped through every channel from one to one hundred and fourteen, stopping at each channel for one count before flipping to the next. After a complete round, I settled to watch what was playing on channel fourteen where three beautiful, thin women were being interviewed about their personal diet and exercise routines. I finished my popcorn and stretched out absolutely mesmerized in awe and envy of their timeless beauty. If I could look even half as good as any one of them, I thought, drifting off to sleep, I know I would undoubtedly be very happy.

Standing restlessly in a long line-up at the bank the next morning, I again pictured those three women and tried desperately to recall some of their beauty secrets. One woman had spoken about how she could eat all her favourite foods, in however small or large a portion she desired, and not gain a single ounce by purging it all afterwards. Another one of them had said that she took an undisclosed number of laxatives on a regular daily basis to push out any extra unwanted calories from her system, and I distinctly remembered her referring to her laxatives as her daily vitamins. She stated that as routinely as the rest of the world took their vitamins on a daily basis to stay healthy, she took her 'vitamins' to stay thin. I wondered curiously if any of their methods would possibly work for me also, even though just thinking about it made me somewhat nauseous. Although I would give almost anything to look as good as any one of them at Steffanni's wedding, I still had no intention of putting any of their crazy methods into practice. When I ran into Phillip and Melinda on my way out of the bank however, my options proved nonexistent.

"Come on sis," Phillip insisted after hearing my third excuse, "Lunch won't take more than an hour. I never get to see you anymore, and you'll have plenty of time afterwards to run your errands before you're needed at the Café."

Realizing he wasn't going to take no for an answer, I paced the sidewalk while he and Melinda finished with their business in the bank, then reluctantly followed them across the street to their favourite restaurant.

"Wow!" Phillip blurted, taking my jacket as I slid into the booth beside Theresa's carrier seat. "You sure have lost a lot of weight sis."

"I have?"

"Well you sure look like you have. Have you been doing some major dieting lately or something?"

"Not really," I lied, trying to sound casual. "Just exercising regularly again. You know, trying to get in shape for Steffanni's wedding."

"Well you surely don't need to lose any more weight" said Melinda. "Any more and the wind will blow you away."

"Oh yeah Melinda, right," I laughed shrugging my shoulders turning to my niece, tickling her tummy. "Your mom's quite the comedian today isn't she? She's really funny. Yes she is," I teased Theresa who was all smiles and giggles. "Oh yes she is."

After carefully calculating the plausable plate worth of everything on the menu presented to me, I decided to play it safe, and order the garden salad. It was the only logical choice for consumption to ensure I didn't exceed my daily allowance.

"Is that all you are having?" Melinda questioned me. "A salad and a glass of water?"

"Oh, I'm going to have something during my break at work later," I lied, straightening and polishing the cutlery laid out in front of me.

"Nonsense," said Phillip. "You hardly get enough of a break at work for anything more than a cup of coffee and a cookie. You're here to have lunch with us now, so you might as well take advantage while you can. My treat. Besides, I would feel guilty eating a big meal when you are only having a salad."

So that was it. For the first time in seven weeks, I gave in to temptation. When the waitress appeared at our table, I ordered my once upon a time, dining out lunch standard. Within minutes, a large oval plate, heaping with greasy, crispy, golden French fries drenched in rich brown gravy lay beside a gristle filled, mayonnaise smothered, bacon, lettuce, and tomato sandwich, and was set before me. The salty, sweet aroma of what had for so long been to me as forbidden fruit, now rose up from my plate like a serpent baiting its prey. I picked up my fork slowly while catching Melinda's glances as if she seemed more interested in my plate than her own. I stabbed a French fry, slowly lifted it to my lips and that was it. Straightaway I was in a tailspin. I was unable to think. I was unable to comprehend anything. I was incapable of stopping. I had utterly forgotten what nourishment tasted like, how much I loved food, and in that moment, I couldn't have cared less how much it was going to pack the fat pounds on me. In what felt like the blink of an eye, but had been nearly twenty minutes, I cleaned my entire plate. I had in addition downed an entire chocolate milkshake, and also eaten my coleslaw which I never ate, even as a kid, because I didn't like the texture. When the rush was over and it indeed hit me what I had just done, I panicked. I closed my eyes and tried to focus on my breathing. This all had to be just another bad dream. Then Phillip's voice cut through my growing fear, and confirmed this was really happening.

"You must have been hungrier than you thought there sis. I don't think I've ever seen you eat coleslaw before now?"

"Uh .... yeah. I, um .... I guess I was hungry."

When I opened my eyes, I realized that Phillip was now holding Theresa in his arms.. *When had he picked up the baby,* I wondered? *Had I picked her up and passed her to him? Had Melinda?* I shook my head in disbelief. I really couldn't remember. *Why could I not remember?* I scanned quickly around the room looking over the other attended tables in the restaurant. I could only imagine what people who had just witnessed my behaviour must be thinking, and I swear I could hear them telepathically. *No wonder she drinks huge milkshakes, if I were a cow like that I would too! No wonder that booth is tilted, with that much weight on it, I'm surprised it doesn't cave in! Good heavens that girl can eat! Where she finds room to pack it all in with all that other fat is beyond me, she's huge! I didn't know they served hippo's here? What a pig! Moooooo!*

The longer I sat, the louder the voices in my head became.

"I gotta go," I said, jumping up, swiftly grabbing my jacket and purse. I tossed a five dollar bill and a twenty on the table, and bent down giving Theresa a quick kiss on the forehead. "I'll see you guys at mom and dad's soon okay. Thanks for lunch." I turned and dashed out of the restaurant as fast as I could without a glance back.

Once outside, I followed the flow of people crossing the street before I stopped. My breath was shallow, and I was finding it difficult to breathe. My heart was pounding so fast I could feel a tingling sensation going down the left side of my neck and arm, causing them to go numb. *Was I having a heart attack?* I wondered? *Fat people like me are at a higher risk to have a heart attack and stroke,* I thought to myself. After what I'd just done, it would not have surprised me. My head started to spin, swirling a cocktail of guilt, fear, anger, rage and confusion about what I'd done. I ran to the end of the next block and darted into the Edson Public Library. I anxiously asked for the key to the washroom, and locked myself safely inside. *You fool!* The voice in my head whispered as I stood panting in front of the mirror. *How could you have been so stupid? What the hell is wrong with you? Do you have any idea the damage you have just done?* Hot tears flooded over my face, burning my dry skin. *You've blown everything you've been working so hard at to achieve!* I glared at the hopeless woman looking back to me. *You are weak! Nothing but weak!* I hissed. *Weak, weak, weak! I hate you!*

I had to do something, anything. I could increase my exercising and decrease my calories even more, but that still wouldn't remedy the mess I was in now. Numbers and thoughts raced through my mind feeding my dizziness, and I felt like I was going to be sick. I looked up into the mirror and shook my head no, but then nodded yes. *That's it! No. I can't. I shouldn't. I couldn't. Could I?* I looked again to the woman in the mirror, more pitiful now than before. *You have to. Don't you see? You did this to yourself. You don't have any other choice.* I walked into the stall, knelt on the cold tiled floor, and took a deep breath in, letting it out slowly counting to fourteen. *Just this once okay,* the voice reassured me. *Just to correct some of the damage you did. You have no other options and you know that.* It was true. Nothing could be any worse than absorbing all those fat calories and garbage. Not even this. I lifted the toilet seat, took in a breath, stuck two fingers to the back of my throat, gagged, but didn't get sick. After trying it a couple more times without success, I got back up and went back over to the mirror. *You have to do this,* I scolded and pleaded with myself at the same time. *This is the only way to protect yourself from the calories, and undo the damage that you've caused yourself. Now get back in there and fix this!* I dug to the bottom off my purse for an elastic band, and pulled my hair tightly back into a ponytail. I took a paper cup from the small dispenser that hung on the wall above the sink, and guzzled down as many cups of warm water I could. I remembered one of the women in the documentary saying that this helped her to purge after she ate, and I could only hope now it would work for me too. When I went back into the stall and knelt down, I tried using three fingers, not two. This time it worked. I heaved and heaved without stopping until I was sure there was nothing left in me to come up. After a minute, I went back to the sink, rinsed out my mouth, and washed my hands and face. *Good girl,* the voice applauded as I brushed out my hair. *I knew you could do it. Well done.* I zipped up my jacket, and hung my purse over my shoulder as I quietly exited the restroom and returned the key to the desk.

"Are you feeling all right ma'am?" asked the librarian. "You were in there quite a long time?"

"Yes thank you, I'm fine." I stated hoarsely, not looking up feeling her eyes following me. Once outside I breathed in the fresh air deeply allowing it to soothe my throat. Strangely enough, I did feel better. As a matter of fact, I was remarkably feeling stronger than I ever have before. I knew what I had just done was truly disgusting, but somehow it proved empowering too. I was still in control. Also, I was now aware that if I were ever in the situation again, where I was forced to partake of any forbidden food, I now knew how to get rid of it. I could now protect myself from all bad food. Most of it at least.

On my way home from work that evening, I stopped at a local pharmacy and purchased four boxes of laxatives. Like the other women in the documentary said, "Vitamins, just to be on the safe side."

5

It had been raining steadily for two hours, and dark grey clouds still blocked the sun. I pulled my laces tight, zipped my jacket to my chin, tied my hair back in my usual ponytail style, locked my front door, and headed toward the park. I just couldn't wait any longer, and I needed to run. The sidewalks were slippery beneath my rubber soles, and I had to focus on my count just to keep my balance, *two-four-six-eight-ten-twelve-four-teen, two-four-six-eight-ten-twelve-four-teen*. The park was empty less a stray dog prancing at the edge of the duck pond, and I was determined not to miss a beat. By the time I'd reached the bakery downtown, a quarter mile short of my goal, I had to stop just to catch my breath. My shoes and socks were both soaking wet, and I could feel a cold chill working its way up my calves that I knew would later turn to painful spasms. I had only stood there a moment before my eyes were scanning the sticky cakes and pastries behind the bakery window. The sweet scent of freshly baking danishes swirled around me. My saliva glands filled my mouth with water as I imagined biting into each and every one of the pastries. Then I heard my name.

"Jenniffer, hey Jenni, is that you?" my mother's voice called out.

I'm sure I turned around with the guilt ridden face of a child who got caught with their hand in the cookie jar.

"I thought that was you I saw run across the street...." She stopped mid sentence and looked directly at me like she knew exactly what I was thinking, "Are you all right Jenni? You look kind of flushed. What are you doing out here in this weather anyhow? Are you trying to catch a cold? Why aren't you driving, where's your car? Oh never mind that now," she continued in her quick manner. "I'm on my way home. Get in the car, and I'll give you a ride."

The stern gleam in her eye let me know the offer was not open for discussion. I tried to act gracious with "That would be great" and followed her to her van. I gave her some excuse when getting in, about my car needing to be taken to the shop for some repairs, but wasn't sure if she'd heard me. She didn't ask me again what I was doing running out in the rain though, she just rambled on about Sunday's upcoming dinner and how big her new grand-baby was getting. I was still fantasizing about cream cheese danishes. It took me a moment when she turned her van into the grocer's parking lot to realize she was stopping to shop.

"Well aren't you coming in?"

"I'll wait here mom." I had to think of something quick. Anything to keep myself from having to look at all that food. "I'll just slow you with my wet shoes on the floor." My excuse sounded as lame to me as it did to her, and she developed a puzzled look.

"Don't be silly Jenni. You know I hate shopping alone. Besides, you can help me carry."

Inside the store I watched people closely as they gathered their desired foods from the shelves and placed them into carts. I went on a huge silent binge, devouring every box, bag and can of food I passed. At the checkout counter, my eyes scanned each item as did the lasers. They calculated the total cost. I calculated calories and fat grams.

In the van on the way home I felt sick. I hated shopping. I felt like an alcoholic touring a winery, being passed sample after sample of chardonnay and Bordeaux.

"I hope the skies clear up before dinner this weekend," mom's voice interrupted my thoughts. "It is so much nicer when we can all go outside and have dessert and tea on the patio. Don't you agree?"

"Yes, it is. But this weekend? I thought dinner was next weekend."

"No dear, it's this Sunday, the eighteenth. Remember, Phillip and Melinda are going to her parents next weekend. You will be there won't you Jenni? Your father will be so disappointed if you miss another family dinner. Especially on Father's Day."

"Of course," I reassured her, "I'll be there. Dinner is at four-thirty right?"

"As always. Will you need a ride? I can pick you up if you need."

"Pick me up?"

"Unless you think you're car will be ready by then?"

"Oh, right. Um, no, I guess it won't be," I fumbled, trying desperately to keep my lie afloat. "I can't drive it for a few days yet."

"Then I'll come get you on Sunday afternoon around four o'clock, okay?"

"I'll be ready, and thanks for the ride home mom." I waved a quick bye from the door as mom beeped her horn and disappeared down the street. When her van turned out of sight, I ran to my kitchen calendar, and sure enough, I had marked dinner for the next weekend. How could I have made such an error? More importantly, what would I wear? Who else was going to be there? Who would I have to sit beside, across from, what would I be forced to eat? Hot tears blurred my vision, and I ran to my closet. I tossed garment after garment over my bed to the floor. Damn you! I screamed, looking at the oversized figure taunting me from the mirror. *Why don't you call Melinda and ask to borrow her maternity clothes now that she's had the baby? Maybe she has something you can hide those thick thighs under.*

Then I remembered the bakery. I didn't run my last quarter mile this afternoon, and I had to make it up. Especially now I thought, with the impending family dinner upon me. I stepped on my treadmill, set it for a full mile just to be safe, and started counting. I then slipped into a steaming hot bath for twenty minutes, dried off and stepped onto the scale. The numbers flashed higher and higher finally stopping at a horrifying 103 pounds. Only half a kilogram under forty-seven. I shook my head in disgust. Still not good enough. I was five pounds under my original goal, but when I looked in the mirror, it proved I was still too fat. I set a new goal for double digits just under one hundred. If I could get down to ninety-nine pounds, or ninety-eight, just to be safe, then for sure I would be ok. Then I would not be fat. Then I would be happy.

I re-ironed my clothes, and hung each of them neatly back on their color coded hangers in their specifically designated space in the closet. I vacuumed the carpet and stretched out on my bed with my books, pen and paper. I wrote down everything I could remember mom buying for dinner at the grocery store earlier. I wrote down everything else I could think of she might use in the additional cooking and preparation for the Sunday dinner, and beside each I wrote down the calorie counts for each item. After totalling the column I divided it by six figuring that to be the total number of guests. My calculations came to a possible consumption rate of one thousand, four hundred and thirty-eight calories per plate. That was more than my entire weeks allowance now! Totally exhausted, somewhere between panic and helplessness, I drifted off to sleep.

6

It was three-fifty five Sunday afternoon when mom rapped on the door. I grabbed my purse, heaved a sigh of despair while making a grimacing face at my reflection in the glass door, and pulled it open. Somehow I mustered a smile. Thousands of people all over the country were getting ready to sit down and share Father's Day dinner with their families today. Why was this so difficult for me?

"I was going to get you to set the table while I finished getting dinner ready," mom said pointing to the white Ford Tempo parked in the driveway, "Looks like Philip and Melinda are already here, so she may have it done already and you can sit and relax."

I swallowed hard trying to wash down the lump slowly developing in my throat. Relax? I thought. Sure, if it were only that simple.

"Hey good lookin'!" Phillips voice echoed down the hallway toward me.

"Hi Phil, it's good to see you." I said, reciprocating his hug.

"Have you lost more weight again?" He asked.

I pulled away quickly from his embrace with a sharp "No! Of course I haven't."

"Hey calm down sis," he said. "There just doesn't seem to be as much of you to hug as the last time I saw you."

"Well I haven't." I said trying not to sound so defensive. The way everyone was looking at me when I walked into the living room though, I knew it was without much success.

"You do look like you've lost a few pounds' Jenni." Dad spoke, looking away from his newspaper. "But you're lookin' good as ever kid." He smiled, and went back to reading his paper.

Twenty eight years old and he still called me kid. I'd chosen to wear my black and grey knit sheath dress, with my grey heels. I thought the heels would make me taller, and combined with the dark colour, I would look thinner. My theory was either working, or everyone was for some reason, just trying to be nice.

"Where's Melinda? Is she here with the baby?" I asked, quickly trying to change the topic, averting attention away from myself.

"Last I saw, her and the baby were in the kitchen with Steffanni." Phil said.

"I'll go say hi."

Before I made it out of the room, both Melinda and Steffi came in to announce dinner was already on the table. A year ago I would have been hurt that mom didn't need my help as requested, but today instead, I was relieved. Other than a little nauseous when we all gathered in the dining room, I felt surprisingly more calm that I had anticipated. I knew the menu in every count by the ounce, and I had it all well planned. So I thought. Then I sat down.

"Lasagna?" I questioned out loud without realizing.

"Yeah, it was Dad's idea." Whispered Steffanni who sat down beside me.

"I shopped with mom three days ago though. She bought a roast and..."

"Dad thought that because it was his favourite and ours, it would be a nice change. Mom said that with it being his Father's Day dinner, he should have what he wanted so we shopped again yesterday, and put the roast in the freezer for another time."

"Oh."

"What's wrong Jenni? Don't you like lasagna anymore? You look almost sick?"

"Oh I'm fine." I lied. "I just had my heart set on roast beef I guess. That's all."

I couldn't answer any questions about the conversation that took place during dinner. Something about babies sleeping, or not sleeping through the night, and maybe something about baseball. I think anyway. I couldn't say for sure. I was too preoccupied trying to figure out how many calories I was forcing into my body just to save face, and the damage it was going to do if it hadn't started to already. What I did know for certain, was that I set my beginning mark at the bottom of my stomach with two small radishes.

It must have been at least an hour before everyone had finished eating, and mom and Steffanni started clearing the table. With Phil and dad in a serious debate on who would win the next World Series, I seized my chance to escape. I'm not sure if they heard me excuse myself from the table, but dad smiled with an approving nod as I rose from my chair. I swiftly left the room and snuck upstairs to my parents' bedroom where I swung back the door, and darted around the corner into the en-suite bathroom. I immediately turned on the hot water faucet to let it get warm, filled the sink cup to the top with warm water and guzzled it down. I counted to fourteen and repeated the ritual three more times as always. I clipped my hair back with one of moms burettes, washed my hands and knelt onto the floor. Taking in a deep breath, I slowly slid my three middle fingers down the back of my throat as far as I could, wiggling them until I unburdened myself of every calorie I had been forced to consume. When I finally saw remnants of the red radishes I had eaten first, my 'mark' as I called it at the bottom of my stomach, I knew I was safe. As safe as I could be for the time being anyhow. I knew I was going to have to add to my exercises before bed when I got home though, just to be sure and get rid of the calories I had already absorbed that turned into fat. I stood up, flushed the toilet, and grabbed the antibacterial spray mom always kept under the sink. I cleaned the toilet of any tell tale signs, closed the lid, and straightened the bath mat. I rinsed my mouth, washed my hands, splashed cool water over my face and patted it dry. Breathing in deeply the rich scent of vanilla that always embodied mom's towels, I definitely felt much better. Since that day at the library, I had become quite good at emptying myself of unwanted foods and I didn't even have to force it all the time anymore. Sometimes, all I had to do was prepare my mind and will my body to obey on command. My body itself, seemed to know when it should, and shouldn't permit or allow food to stay. I smiled at the strong woman in the mirror with the proud look of success, and brushed out my hair. "See, you got through dinner ok, and you did just fine." I said out loud, placing mom's brush back into the drawer. "Now all you have to do is get through dessert, and you'll be home free."

"And how would you like that dessert Jenniffer? At the table, or preferably in the bowl?"

I turned and suddenly froze on the spot like Lot's wife had looking behind at the forbidden city, only my heart left pounding. I had snuck up the stairs and into the bathroom so hurriedly, I'd neglected to check the bedroom when I ran through. Melinda had been lying on the bed feeding the baby, and now she was standing in the doorway beside me with a sheer look of horror and disgust.

7

I took in a slow deep breath and got my bearings. "Oh, hi. Did you say something?" I asked as casually as I could. "Do you need to use the bathroom?"

"Don't play dumb with me Jenniffer, I know what you are doing. I just heard you throw up all your supper!"

I didn't speak. I just glared at her wondering exactly how long she had actually been there watching me. How dare she invade my privacy like this!

"Well? Are you going to say something or are you just going to stand there with that oh so innocent look on your face?"

"I don't understand what you mean," I said acting totally unaware. I knew I had to remain calm and focussed. Melinda was no fool.

"Is this some new ritual you perform after you eat now? The cause of all this weight you've lost?"

"What?" I laughed. "I'm sorry, but I really don't know what you are talking about."

"Oh really now?" She said accusingly.

"Really," I insisted. "I've had a stomach flu for a few days now. The spices and garlic just didn't sit well with me tonight. That's all."

"Oh I see. So I'm supposed to believe that hearing you making yourself sick was all in my mind?"

"I don't know what you think you heard Melinda, but if that's what you think, I assure you that you are wrong."

"And I suppose you congratulating yourself for throwing up was all my imagination too?"

I could feel my body start to tremble with anger. She wasn't buying anything I said, and it was obvious that she wasn't going to let me get away from her that easily either. I tried to walk past her and the baby, but she put her free arm out to block the door.

"You're not going anywhere until I am finished with this Jenniffer."

"You are more than finished," I growled back at her. She only dropped her arm when mom walked around the corner.

"What's going on up here? You two aren't arguing are you? I could hear voices half way down the stairs." Mom said.

"Ask her," I huffed, shaking my head while pushing my out of the room between them. "She's totally crazy!"

The rest of the evening was a complete nightmare. Melinda kept watching my every move. She served me my dessert herself despite my said upset stomach, and then followed me to the kitchen to return my plate. There was no escaping to a bathroom without her shadowing me for a minute. Mom kept looking at me with this quizzing look smiling, and then to Melinda questionably. The scrutiny was becoming unbearable. When Steffanni announced she was leaving, I immediately volunteered her services to drop me off at my place. A very long two hours later I was finally home free, safely comforted within the privacy of my own walls.

The next few days I sacrificed my daily jog for extra miles on my treadmill, and took some additional time off work. I turned the ringer off on both telephones and unplugged my answering machine. I didn't want to see anyone, but most important I didn't want to be seen. I chased the unending guilt from dessert at my parent's place with my entire month's supply of laxatives, swallowing them fourteen at a time with bottles of mineral oil. I was determined to flush out every rotten calorie if it killed me in the process. And it was. Totally unaware, little by little my body deteriorated, feeding itself on it's own muscle and organ tissue alone. The pain it caused me was excruciating, but also exhilarating. To me it meant that I was winning the war against my fat, and that gave me renewed strength. I exercised in two hour intervals and slept in between when I could.

By the end of the second week in seclusion, I felt strong and powerful, once again ready to face the world outdoors.

8

The days and nights had passed quickly undetermined within the sanctuary of my own home. I hadn't spoken to anyone but Ken and Marianne since Father's Day, so it shouldn't have surprised me when mom and Melinda showed up on my front doorstep. I raced through the kitchen and living room doing a fast tidy before unlocking the door to let them in, then rushed back to my room to change my clothes. I called out saying I'd be right there, and quickly slipped from my pyjamas into my powder blue jogging suit before meeting them in the hall.

"Hi guys, what brings you two to this side of town?" I warbled.

"We stopped in at the restaurant for lunch to see you, and Janice said you hadn't been at work for days now," began Melinda. "Your mother has called here a few times and you haven't returned any of her calls either. Frankly, we've all become very concerned about you Jenniffer."

"Concerned, Why?" I asked making light of her tone, smiling. "I've just been off sick with some flu or something. You knew I hadn't been feeling well."

"Jenni you look absolutely terrible," mom spoke. "Are you sure it's just the flu? Have you seen a doctor?"

"I'll be fine Mom, really. Whatever it is will have run its course soon, and I'll be feeling better before you know it. No reason to worry I am sure."

"Well as long as we're here now, we might as well stay and share a pot of tea with you before we go," said Melinda. "You don't mind company for awhile do you Jenniffer? I think we all could use some sustenance."

"Why would I mind?" I lied not amused by her ambush. "I was just going to make a cup of tea for myself before the doorbell rang."

Since mom insisted I rest while she got the tea, I sat at the table with Melinda not speaking a word. I didn't have to be looking toward her to know she was watching me. I could feel her obstinate stare.

"What are those odd looking spots on your sweatshirt Jenniffer?" She asked scrunching her face. "It looks like you've spilled something but the spots look like they keep expanding."

I looked down at my sleeves puzzled. There was a wet patch on my shoulder and a couple more becoming largely visible on my left arm.

"Oh shit! Uhh, it must be water," I replied quickly. "I was washing dishes a few minutes ago and probably splashed myself or something. You know how clumsy I can be," I said standing up. "I'll go change and be right back. I'll only be a minute."

I couldn't believe how easy it was becoming to lie. I didn't even have to think anymore. I just opened my mouth and the words flowed spontaneously. It was the physical cover-ups that were proving difficult.

Back in my bedroom I grabbed a black, long sleeved shirt and sweater on my way past the closet to my bathroom, then stripped off my soiled clothing and threw it all under the sink.

Speak of bad timing. The two bottles of mineral oil I had just
guzzled for lunch had begun seeping through my skin, soaking
into my cotton track suit. I had to move quickly not to arouse any
suspicion, so I towelled off the best I could, and smoothed a thin
layer of corn starch and baby powder over my arms and bodice
before redressing, hoping it wouldn't happen again.

Going back down the hall I could hear mom and Melinda
talking, their voices in a low whisper.

"I can understand why you don't want to believe there is
anything really wrong Victoria. If it were my child, I wouldn't want
to believe it either. Regardless, you have to think of what's best
for Jenniffer right now. Honestly, I believe that whatever it is
causing her to resort to these not only unusual, but dangerous
behaviours, it needs outside attention that none of us are
equipped to give her."

"What, you mean? Like a psychiatrist?"

"Maybe it wouldn't be a bad idea."

"My daughter is not crazy Melinda. She is just....."

"Just what Victoria? Jogging excessively in the cold rain?
Starving herself into thin air? Forcing herself to throw up every
scrap of food she actually might put into her mouth?"

"Now stop it! That's enough! You don't know that she is
doing that purposely. You are only speculating."

"I heard and saw her with my own two ears and eyes Victoria!"
She emphasized. "It was like watching someone perform some
kind of ritual. Planned, premeditated, and precise."

"I think you are reading way too much into things Melinda.
She explained what you heard and saw."

"She made excuses for what I saw and heard. The same way she is making excuses for her absence and behaviour now."

They were quiet for a moment, and then Melinda walked over to my fridge and opened it.

"Look," she said holding the refrigerator door wide open, peering inside. "There is nothing in here except for mouldy bread, skim milk, some condiments, and dried up leftovers she brought from your place almost two weeks ago now. It's completely untouched and still in the container you sent it in. Why, I'll bet she hasn't eaten anything all week, maybe even since then for that matter."

"She has been ill. You see how sick she is."

"She is making herself sick!"

"That's enough Melinda. I'm telling you that you are over exaggerating and that Jenniffer is going to be just fine once she is over this flu. Now we are not discussing this again. Do you understand what I am saying?"

"I understand that you are in denial."

I walked abruptly around the corner before mom could reply any further. I myself had listened to more than enough.

"Who is in denial about what?" I questioned, trying to sound unknowingly and casual.

They both looked up. Mom with a concerned sympathetic eye; Melinda completely overthrown by her. It looked good on Melinda too I thought. She had no right invading my personal life the way she had, and mom had every right to put her in her place for doing so.

"Nothing dear," mom replied hesitantly, summoning a smile. "We were just talking."

I poured myself a cup of tea, adding milk and two cubes of sugar to try and make it look good. I went to the pantry and took out a box of plain cookie biscuits I'd purchased a couple months back. I placed fourteen cookies on a saucer and centred it on the table. I then took two cookies for myself, and sneered at Melinda.

An hour and a half later, and they finally decided it was time to leave. I assured mom with a hug that I would call her if I needed anything, and that I would make a doctor's appointment and get checked out if I wasn't feeling better within the next couple of days. I waited until they had completely turned out of the driveway and waved goodbye, before closing and locking the door behind them. *Why did they have to stay so long? Why did they come over in the first place? Damn that Melinda,* I thought on my way back to the kitchen to clean up. *It was all her idea to come here in the first place and I just knew it. Why couldn't she just mind her own damn business for once? At least mom seemed to believe my stories over hers which gave me some reprieve.* I chuckled at the recollection of Melinda's face when mom finally told her to shut up.

Then I saw the empty tea cups and remembered the cookies, the milk, and worst of all, the sugar cubes. I ran to my bathroom as fast as I could. The dirty dishes would have to wait.

9

Curled tightly in a fetal position, I awoke lying in the middle of the carpet on my bathroom floor, trembling like a long blade of grass on a windy day. Buried under my housecoat and a towel I must have pulled over myself at some point, I tried to focus my thoughts. Everything was a haze. I couldn't remember why I was lying there, or how long I had been there. I was shivering from the cold, and tried to push myself to my feet but couldn't find the strength. At my every attempt to get up, my legs buckled under me like a newborn fawn trying to stand for the first time, and pain shot from my ankles straight to the top of my spine. Eventually I gave up trying to stand, and let myself curl back down into the shaggy carpet. If it hadn't been so difficult to breathe I would have cried. Exhausted, I silently counted the gold flecks on the ceiling tiles above my left shoulder until sleep thankfully took hold again.

"Jenniffer! Jenniffer, wake up!" I heard mom yelling frantically, while shaking my arm. "What are you doing in here laying in the middle of the floor?"

I half opened my eyes and looked up. I tried so hard to speak, but my voice was trapped somewhere in my throat. My tongue was completely dry, and stuck to the bottom of my chapped mouth. I recognized my mom standing over me, but I couldn't make out the hazy figure behind her until she spoke.

"Is she okay mom?"

"I don't know Steffanni," Mom answered. "She's been so sick lately. Run out to the car and get the baby. Tell Melinda to come right in and help me. Please, hurry!"

Mom knelt down and lifted my housecoat with intentions of getting me up. When Steffanni and Melinda came in, they found her still on the floor beside me, sobbing, shaking her head back and forth with both hands clasped over her mouth.

"Good heavens Victoria! What's happened?"

Melinda's voice tangled with my sisters, then trailed off somewhere in the distance as I drifted in and out of consciousness. I was ninety-two pounds now, and looking down at me, the three of them could easily see each one of my ribs individually, protruding back to front like a rack of lamb on a spit. My legs and arms had become like sticks on a marionette, and a soft layer of fine hair covered my dry skin that was cracked and flaked like dandruff. When I awoke next, I was laying on my sofa in the living room, under a big woollen blanket, now dressed in a dry warm flannel gown. Mom was at my side holding my hand gently in hers.

"Jenni, can you hear me?" she asked in a quiet voice.

I nodded, forcing a weak smile.

"Can you tell me what happened? When I came in, I found you collapsed on your bathroom floor."

"I .... I'm not sure." I mumbled.

"I was so scared when I saw you laying there not moving," Steffanni blurted out. "You looked like you were dead!"

Mom snapped her head around quickly toward my sister who was sitting at my feet. "Don't you ever say that again Steffanni, do you hear me?"

The air was suddenly still, heavy with emotion. My sisters' face saddened in a way I had never seen before as mom kept her unbroken glare. Melinda walked over and put her arm around Steffanni's shoulder when my sister started to cry, and motioned her toward the kitchen.

"Come on Steffi," she said, "Let's go and make some tea and leave the two of them alone to talk."

After they'd gone, mom turned back to me and smiled.

"Can I get you anything Jenni?"

"I think the furnace is broken," I said weakly.

"What makes you think that?"

"It's so cold."

"It's over eighty degrees in here," she stated quizzically. "If anything, it is much too warm. Honestly honey, I don't know how you can find it cold at all."

"Oh." was all I replied, and slid myself further under the heavy blanket tucked around me. I was fully awake now, and remarkably alert.

"Jenniffer, I want you to be honest with me about some things," Mom spoke tenderly. "I want you to tell me if Melinda has been right about you all this time. About what you have been doing to yourself. I want you to know I will help you however I can, but first you have to be completely honest with me okay." She paused. "Have you been the one lying to me Jenniffer?"

Shocked by her frankness, I locked my eyes with hers, searching for some sign of hope that I could still make her believe me. A part of me longed to tell her everything. About how it all started with a simple diet to lose a few pounds. About how Cindy had cautioned me about the dangers ahead of me if I carried on dieting to such extremes. About how losing control made me feel in fact more in control, and how empty I had become not just physically from the lack of food, but emotionally from life itself. I wanted to scream and cry out to Mom for help right then in that moment to save me from this hell. I wanted to beg for her forgiveness for being such a horrible daughter and genuinely promise never to lie to her again. More than all of that though, still, a bigger part of me, the fat part of me, needed to keep my secrets. I still needed to be thinner.

"Lying to you about what mom?" I asked. "Just what exactly has Melinda been telling you?"

"You honestly don't know?" She asked me, our eyes deadlocked.

"Look Mom, if Melinda has been saying things about me, or I'm being accused of something, I think it's only fair that I am given the courtesy of knowing what it is. Don't you?"

"Well honey, Melinda is convinced that the reason you are sick and have lost so much weight is because you are purposely trying to."

I shook my head. "I don't understand. I was exercising again to get in better shape for Steffi's wedding, but then I caught this flu. I told you that mom. I told her too."

"Yes, that's true, but Melinda thinks you've been lying about the flu. She thinks it's more than that."

"Like what exactly?"

"Melinda thinks that you have been refraining from eating, and then forcing yourself to throw it all back up when you do eat."

"That's awful," I said almost in a whisper, breaking our eye contact. "That is so disgusting."

"Yes it is," she agreed. "But is it true Jenniffer?"

"What? Why would I want to make myself sick like that mom? Why would anyone?"

I absolutely hated myself for lying to her, but I had no other choice. More and more she was doubting me and believing that nosy sister in law of mine. I had to somehow divert attention back to Melinda, and make her look like the crazy one.

"Mom," I said in a low whisper, "Do you think it's possible that Melinda could be suffering from some sort of postpartum depression or something. Should we need to be concerned about her? Maybe she should be the one to see a doctor. Why else would she think and say such horrible things about me?"

"I don't know Jenni. That's the part I can't figure out myself." She reached over and slid a strand of hair that had fallen over my face back behind my ear, and her eyes started welling with tears. "You are so very thin honey. So frail."

"Please don't cry Mom. Please," I begged. "I'm not trying to make myself sick. Honest. I'm not."

"But you've have lost so much weight Jenni," she emphasized again.

"Not really," I shrugged. "Just a couple of pounds for the wedding. It probably just looks like more 'cause I'm pale from this flu. I might be a little dehydrated though but really, that's all."

"A little dehydrated? Jenniffer look at your hair. You had such beautiful hair not so long ago, and now it's not only dry and brittle, but it's falling out around you. Now really, that is not symptomatic of the flu."

"No. No you're right. It's not. But what happened with my hair is that, well, you see, I tried to do one of those home permanents a couple nights ago... and... and well... I confused the waving lotion with the pre-perm conditioner. Can you believe it? The lotion was on my hair the entire two hours it took me to roll the curlers before I realized that I'd even done it. That's why my hair is so awful the way it is now."

"Well why on earth would you try and do a home permanent all by yourself? If you'd called and asked, you know I would have come over and helped you."

"I know mom, and I did think of that, but it was just one of those impulse things when I was at the pharmacy to pick up some cold medicine, and I was anxious to get it done. You know how I can be. I just purchased the box, came back home and next thing you know... Well you can see for yourself the results."

Mom didn't say anything. She just sat staring blankly at me, as if looking right through me as clearly as a pane of glass. My lies were becoming too transparent. I knew I had gone too far now, yet couldn't stop. Still determined to convince her that my story was the truth, I went for the compassionate sympathy plea.

"I just wanted to do something to try and pick myself up a bit after feeling so lousy lately. Try a little change."

I looked down, and pouted like I did when I was a little girl. She always gave in to that. "I thought trying some new hairstyles for Steffanni's wedding would be fun, and well... do you think it will grow back out in time for the wedding? Can you maybe help me try and fix it Mom?"

Steffanni walked back into the living room carrying Theresa, and Melinda followed close behind them with a tea tray before mom could reply any further.

"We have come up with a great idea," Melinda said while handing me a cup of tea she no doubt had dumped a pound of sugar into. "Steffanni and I were talking in the kitchen and we think that you should go back and stay at home for a few days until you get well again Jenni. Just in case you have another falling down incident that is."

"Oh now I think that is a fabulous idea!" Mom exploded, breaking into a smile.

"Yeah, you can stay in your old room, and you can help me with wedding plans and things," Steffanni beamed. "We'll have so much fun Jenni. Please say yes," she begged. "It will be just like old times again."

"Oh I .... I don't know," I stuttered, trying not to sound as panicked as I suddenly felt. "Don't you think I would probably be more in the way than any kind of real help to you? Besides, I don't want anyone else to catch whatever this flu that I have is."

"Don't be silly," Mom insisted standing up. "Not only is it a great idea, but it is already settled. I'll go pack up a bag with some of your things for a few days stay, and you rest here and finish your tea."

"No!" I screamed loudly, and all three of them jerked, completely taken aback by my outburst.

"What do you mean no?" Mom questioned in an agitated tone that let me know instantly, there was nothing I could do to get out of this one.

"I.... I just mean no, that I can get up and go pack my own things." I set down my cup and got to my feet as they all watched me suspiciously. "You all stay here and finish your tea," I insisted. "I know where everything I will need is, and we can be ready to go a lot quicker if I do it myself. Besides, I can't exactly go out in my nightgown, so I have to change."

I made my way down the hall to my bedroom, leaving my mother and sister with Melinda the brainwashing ringleader, again free to conspire against me in my absence. Well at least I had successfully averted drinking that tea I thought, tossing random things into my suitcase. The next few days however, were going to be a much bigger challenge. With mom catering to my so called needs, it was going to make sticking to my diet extremely difficult, and any exercise almost impossible. Then there was Melinda. She undoubtedly would be circling my parents' house constantly watching me like a hawk fixed on her own personal prey.

10

My bedroom was almost the same as I'd left it seven years before. The powder blue wallpaper with textured lilacs mom and I spent two days hanging when I was sixteen, still clung tightly to the walls. A soft lilac carpet covered the floor, and flat white paint finished the borders and ceiling. My old wooden bed and dresser, handed down to me after Phillip moved out of the house, remained where I had left them. Although now somewhat faded, my old light blue, satin comforter ensemble still matched the room perfectly. The only real change mom had made to the room was a pair of new white shears over the window, and her sewing table now sat under the window where my makeup table used to sit. When I took in a deep breath, I could still detect the scent of lavender lingering from the hundreds of incense sticks I had burned in my room over the years. I walked over to my old dresser and pulled open the top left hand drawer. Sure enough, two old lavender sticks and a charred incense burner rolled to the front of the drawer. In some ways I guess it was comforting to be back in my old room where I grew up, and I questioned if I'd never left home, if maybe I wouldn't have become so fat living on my own? *Why did I get so fat in the first place*, I wondered? *And when did I get so fat? For that matter, what if I had been fat all my life, and just no-one told me?* I shut the dresser drawer and lay down on my bed. The satin was soft and inviting. I pulled a pillow out from under the sheets and placed it between my knees to keep them from bruising. *Maybe I would stay here for just a few days to do some research into my past,* I thought. I was going to have to dig out the old family photos and slides to see just how fat I was as I grew up, and see if I could find any indications as to when it started. I closed my eyes, and stretched my arms straight out from my sides to the edge of the bed, trying to remember how much of the bed I actually took up at each age of my life. Somewhere between twelve and thirteen I lost track, and fell asleep.

When I woke, I wasn't sure how long I had slept, but thought it must have been at least a couple of hours. However long, it wasn't long enough. I still felt exhausted. I knew I should get up, do the polite thing and go thank Mom for allowing me to come home and rest while I'm "ill" as my so loving sister in law put it. And too, I wanted to let her know that except still a little tired, I was already feeling much better, and wouldn't be staying more than a couple of days. Three or four if I absolutely had to in order to keep the peace, at the most. The more I actually thought about getting up, the lazier I seemed to get. The truth was, I was not in the socializing mood at all, and I wasn't really feeling all that gracious for the coerced invitation home either. I was still very angry with Melinda and extremely frustrated. All I really needed was to be back in my own apartment where I could do what I had to do without anyone else bothering me. Instead though, now I was here trapped in my parents' home, forced to keep up the charade of having the flu.

"You're awake," Steffanni said, peeking around the half opened bedroom door.

"Yeah, I'm up," I said rubbing my eyes, yawning. "How long was I out for? Is dad home from work yet?"

"Home? Only since last night! Jenni, it's Saturday evening. You've been crashed out for practically two whole days now."

"What? No. Two days? I couldn't be."

"Oh yes you have been." Steffanni said, sitting down on the bed beside me as I pushed myself up. "Sis, can I ask you something?" she said without looking at me. "I mean, without you getting mad at me, or taking it the wrong way?"

I reached out and took her hand. "You know you can ask me anything Steffi. What is it?"

She didn't answer, but I could tell something was really bothering her. "Is everything okay with you and Richard?" I asked her. "You didn't have a fight did you? There isn't a problem with the wedding is there?"

When Steffanni finally looked up at me, she had the same blank look on her face that I remembered Mom having when questioning me at my place.

"Richard and I .... the wedding .... everything is fine. I have no concerns with any of that. It's you that I'm worried about."

"Me? Why on earth are you worried about me? I'll be fine once I get over this damn flu."

"But that's just what concerns me Jenni. You say that you will be fine, but obviously something is definitely not right with you. You say you have a flu or something right, but Melinda says...."

"I thought I heard voices," Dad interrupted, entering my room.

"Hi Dad," I said trying to sound cheerful.

"You had us a little worried there Sleeping Beauty," he said. "We were just about to send out the horseman to find you a prince charming and wake you!"

"Oh Daddy," I laughed, embracing his warm hug.

"You my princess are pining away. If you don't get well soon and gain some weight back, there won't be anything left of you."

Steffanni and I exchanged glances.

"Are you feeling any better at all?" Dad asked. "From what your mother tells me, she found you in pretty rough shape the other day."

"I'm actually feeling a lot better Dad," I said yawning again. "I think all I needed was a good couple days rest."

"Good. That's my girl," he said patting my knee, then heading back to the door. "Your mother will be pleased to hear it too. I'll let her know you're up, and to set your place at the table for you. She should have dinner ready in about half an hour."

Steffanni must have recognized the panic in my eyes when dad mentioned dinner. As soon as he shut the door, she turned and looked me straight in the eyes.

"Okay that does it. Now I know something is wrong," she demanded. "So what gives? And I want the truth, so don't say it's nothing."

I didn't say anything because in that moment I didn't know what to say. Steffanni and I had always been so close. Growing up we had shared everything. Our age difference had never been a problem and only seemed to bond us closer. We were not only sisters, but best friends from the day mom and dad brought her home from the hospital. We were so tight that people were always joking with Mom that she had had a set of twins, only seven years apart. She always joked back about us giving her seven years of hard labour. Steffanni and I were nothing but inseparable. We never hid anything, or kept any secrets from each other, mostly because we couldn't. The other sister always knew when something wasn't right. Even after I'd moved into my own place, Steffanni and I would talk for hours over the telephone every evening about our day. It has only been since setting her wedding date that we haven't been as communicative. Understandably though, she has been busy with all the arrangements, and I have been busy with my diet.

"Is it something at work that has got you so upset you're not eating?" Steffanni asked. "You know, you don't have to stay at the Café if you don't want to. You can still go back to school if that's what you want. You know. You're still young enough, regardless what anyone else thinks, and you don't have any kids or anyone at home to worry about."

"It's not work," I said.

"Then it is my wedding that has got you so upset, isn't it?"

I pulled a blanket up to cover my fat body. *Could she really know*, I wondered?

"We always said that if one of us found love before the other, that we'd wait to get married, and have a double wedding. That's it, isn't it Jenni?" She continued. "I should have known when daddy joked about that too, and now everyone's teasing you about still being single, when I am the youngest and getting married in a few months. I should have guessed."

A few months? If the wedding was still a few months away, I could easily lose the weight I needed to. It was only a few weeks now. To lose the weight I needed to I had only eleven weeks left!

"Don't be ridiculous Steffi." I insisted. "It's not that at all. You know as much as I do that you and Richard would be rolling down the isle in wheelchairs if you waited for me to have our dream double wedding. Besides, we swore a lot of things when we were younger, and I don't expect all of them will come to pass."

"What? You mean we're not going to be Bond girls and win an Oscar?" She chuckled.

"Or Dallas Cowboy Cheerleaders!" I whooped, smacking her over the head with my pillow.

"But Richard will be so heartbroken," she feigned. "I was going to give him a calendar for an anniversary present next year!"

Steffanni and I laughed so hard we cried, and it felt so good to spend time with her again, that I actually forgot for a moment what it was that had brought me back here in the first place. Then mom knocked on the door.

"I hate to break up the party girls, but dinner's ready."

11

I slowly followed Steffanni downstairs to the dining room. I knew she was still talking to me, giggling about something else we played at in childhood, but I was no longer interested in any of what she was saying. All I cared about now, was getting through another family dinner. When I sat down, Dad was already heavily buttering a warm crescent bread roll.

"You must be starving kiddo," he said reaching over, placing the buttered roll onto my plate. "You can start with that. How does that old saying go Mother," he continued. "Feed a cold and starve a fever, or is it starve a cold and feed a fever? Whichever, we've got to fatten you up kiddo, so you can get better, and gain your strength back."

"I've been in the kitchen making some of your favourites since I heard you were up," Mom said passing me a pot of steaming hot gravy. "Have as much of whatever you like, or a little of everything if you wish. I have a strawberry rhubarb pie in the oven for dessert too, so save some room."

I looked the table over anxiously looking for anything that I could eat that would satisfy everyone without destroying me in the process. If I had actually slept as long as Steffanni said I had, I could allow myself about three hundred calories safely I thought. The roll Dad so generously put on my plate already surpassed that by far. I poured myself a cup of tea and grabbed a lemon from the fruit bowl. Stalling, I carefully cut it into fourteen even wedges, and squeezed one wedge into my tea.

"Surely now, that isn't all you are having?" Dad asked sounding highly annoyed by my behaviour. "Pass your sister the Linguini Steffanni. Sick or not, I've never known anyone in this family to ever pass on your Mother's linguini and shrimp sauce."

I have no way out, I thought to myself, desperately holding back my tears. *I'm trapped again, and I've got to break my diet. It isn't fair! It's my body, and I should be the one to say when I eat, and when I don't. I should also be the one to say what I eat for that matter, and not forced to eat linguini and bread rolls when I don't want to. Here Jenniffer, eat some pie, eat some butter, dump a bag of sugar into your tea! Why did I ever give Mom that key to my apartment? Why did this damn fat ugly body of mine have to betray me the same day she came over? Why, Why, Why? Why can't I just be thin and be a normal person?* I was so angry I didn't realize I was shovelling enormous amounts of food into my mouth with every thought. I had finished the roll, a full plate of linguini, and was halfway through a thick slice of pork roast, dripping with gravy when I became aware I had lost all control and done it again. I put down my knife and fork, and picked up my still full cup of tea. *What the hell was I doing? Did I not have even a shred of self discipline or willpower left in me at all? How could I keep letting this happen over and over again? And why when it did, was I so unaware of doing it?* I gulped down my tea without stopping for a breath, and excused myself from the table. I thanked Mom for going to such efforts preparing such a wonderful dinner, and had to promise both her and Dad that I would come back down later for a slice of pie. I'd have to find a way to get out of that later by pretending to have fallen asleep or something. Right now though, I had to get rid of the food I'd again so gluttonously devoured. I started to add up the calories and fat grams I'd swallowed as I walked up the stairs, but stopped. I was terrified to know. I knew enough that it must be in the thousands, and if I didn't get rid of it soon, I would weigh a tonne by morning.

I didn't want to risk using Mom and Dad's en-suite again after being caught last time, and the main bathroom was directly across the hall from mine and beside Steffanni's. If Steffanni went into her bedroom she would no doubt hear me if I threw up, and I couldn't take the risk of having to dodge more prying questions. I went back downstairs and told Mom and Steffanni that I was going to go have a shower to freshen up, and that I would be back down after awhile. It was a good story I thought, and seemed to go over without any suspicion. If there was one thing I had always been infamous in this house for it was taking extra long, very hot showers. Tying up the bathroom for a lengthy period of time now would not seem anything out of the ordinary. I turned on the hot water and let it run until steam fogged over everything and filled the room. I didn't want to see any part of my disgusting reflection in any of the chrome or mirrors. After standing under the hot stream of water long enough to warm my naked body, I began to purge. Hopefully any noise was drowned out by the pulsating noise of the showerhead. Unsure of how much I had actually consumed, and what mark I had set if I even had, I couldn't stop myself. When I looked down and noticed traces of blood pooling around the drain, I finally gave up. The sight of blood at one time used to stir something in me that made me feel a little uneasy, and for a moment question whether or not something was wrong. Nowadays it was happening so frequently, I felt it more of a reassurance that my stomach was again empty. In the moment, the sight of blood seemed like it was a good thing, and I actually would have worried more if I didn't see it, meaning there was still a calorie left in me. That thought terrified me more than anything else. I cleaned the tub, allowing the water to run until it drained freely without attention, and then stepped out. Knowing that the laxatives I had hidden in my suitcase would flush any extra calories from my system that remained, I finally started to relax. I toppled my hair on top of my head with a small hand towel, and wrapped a bath sheet around me three times to keep it up before tucking it in. Tidying up the bathroom, I was glad the mirror was still fogged over. Although Mom's towels used to only wrap around me twice, I still didn't want to see my reflection and the fat hanging over the towel I knew was still there.

I scurried across the hall back to my room to find my suitcase wasn't beside my dresser where I'd originally placed it, nor had it been put in my closet. I crouched down to look under my bed but alarmingly it wasn't there either. When I stood up, Steffanni was standing in my doorway making strange faces and gestures. She looked like she was trying to say something but had just had her tongue cut off and couldn't.

"What?" I asked sharply. "Why are you looking at me like that?"

Steffanni remained silent, but it was obvious she really wanted to speak.

"Oh for heaven's sake Steffi, what the hell is it? Can't you see I'm a little busy right now?"

"Busy? B..b...busy?" She finally spit out. "Doing what? Counting your bones?"

I stared at her, completely stunned by her outburst.

"Um, no. I am trying to find my suitcase for your information, so I can get dressed into some clean clothes and go help Mom with the dishes."

Steffanni walked over to my dresser and pulled open the top drawer. "Here," she said in a strangely cold tone of voice, "Mom put all your clothes away in the dresser while you were sleeping, and you can find your empty suitcase on the top shelf of the hall closet."

I stomped out of my room without giving Steffanni a second glance, and opened the closet. With one hand I held up my towel, and with the other I pulled down my suitcase. Setting it down right there on the hallway carpet, I flipped it open and ran my fingers over the dark bottom lining. My secret compartment had been emptied.

"What's wrong now Jenni? Can't find your little pink pills?"

I tipped back the suitcase and searched again.

"Are you going through withdrawal now that you are back in the land of the living or what?" Steffanni continued sarcastically. "Not that you look like you are in the land of the living that's for sure. You look more like a walking skeleton from the land of the living dead."

"Shut up!" I screamed at her. "Just shut the hell up!"

"Why should I? Does the truth hurt that much sis?"

I stood up and shoved my suitcase back into the closet and slammed the door, turning to face her.

"Melinda has told me everything that you've been doing you know." Steffanni shook her head side to side. "Boy is she ever right on the money too. She has you pegged to a tee. Right down to this little panic attack you're having over your laxatives, or rather your 'vitamins' as you have them carefully re-labelled."

"You don't know a damned thing. And neither does Melinda." I cried.

"Well obviously she does!" Steffanni yelled back to me.

I tried to grab my pills out of Steffanni's hand, but she pulled back.

"All I ever hear from any of you anymore is Melinda says this, Melinda says that! I thought sisters of all people were supposed to stick together and support one another, not turn on each other and side with their nosy sister-in-law's crazy tales of fiction!"

"Hey girls," Mom hollered from the bottom of the stairs. "What's all the shouting up there about?"

"Nothing!" I screamed, spinning around. "And I'm not eating dessert! I'm not staying here either! I'm leaving right now and going back home to my own apartment where I can have some privacy!"

I must have spun too quickly when I turned because although I knew my feet weren't moving, my body and everything around me seemed to be in slow motion. I could see Mom's lips moving and knew she was speaking, but I couldn't hear her voice. All I could hear was a high pitched humming sound somewhere in the back of my head. Then suddenly, I felt free; weightless as if I was falling down a deep hole like the one Alice in Wonderland fell into while chasing a white rabbit. My entire body went numb. I couldn't feel anything. I couldn't see anything through the darkness, and I couldn't hear anything but the humming sound getting softer and softer seemingly farther and farther away. The black hole that had enveloped me was so peaceful, and every part of me felt so light, that in that exact moment, I wondered if this was what it felt like to be dying.

12

"I think she's coming around," a voice echoed somewhere around me. I slowly blinked open my eyes, trying to focus on my surroundings.

"Mom?" I whispered.

"No dear. She will be back shortly. My name is Nurse Campbell."

A nurse? Where was I, and how did I end up here? I tried to sit up, but an overwhelming sharp pain shot through my chest forcing me back down, and a warm hand pressed firmly down on my shoulder.

"You just lay back and relax dear. We don't want you to cause any further damage now do we?"

"Damage?" I moaned, trying desperately to find a comfortable position that didn't hurt quite so much. "You make me sound like a train wreck or something."

"Ahh, your sister has a sense of humour I see," Nurse Campbell said to another figure approaching.

"Steffanni? Is that you?" I whispered, unable to breathe in too deeply due to the pain in my chest.

"Yes it's me," she said taking my hand gently into hers. "How are you feeling?"

"It hurts to talk. Where am I?"

"I'll go page the Doctor now that you're awake," Nurse Campbell said. "I will see if I can get him to order something for your pain."

"Thank you," Steffanni said, and I heard a heavy door swing shut. "Mom went to the cafeteria to get something to eat. I've got some water and ice chips here if you want some? The doctor said when you woke up we should try to get you to drink something. Are you thirsty?"

I shook my head no, and looked around, trying to put the pieces together.

"I'm in the hospital, aren't I Steffi?" She nodded. "But why? I mean, how did I get here?"

"You don't remember?" She asked.

And I didn't. Not at first anyway. I knew I must have passed out again though, and in the future I thought, making a mental note to myself, I must be more cautious. My fainting spells were happening all too frequently.

"It's all my fault!" Steffanni cried, her face suddenly flooding with tears as if a dam just broke behind her eyes. "I'm so sorry Jenni! If I hadn't been so mean and yelled at you, you wouldn't have fallen." She looked at me sadly and somewhat confused. "You really don't remember, do you? My gosh Jenni, you looked like a rag doll I had just tossed down the stairs to mom's feet."

I didn't remember fighting with Steffanni. I did remember having a sense of her being some kind of threat to me in some way though, however I couldn't remember why or how. I then remembered the darkness too that when surrounding me, gave me a euphoric sense of lightness and freedom. I closed my eyes. *If I could have only one wish right now,* I thought to myself, *it would be to be back in there, in that black hole where there was no fear or pain and being fat didn't matter.* Tuning in to Steffanni's voice again, I reopened my eyes.

"Now you're laying here all broken up and it's all my fault." she sobbed. "I'm sorry I said all those horrible things to you Jenni. I wasn't trying to hurt you, honestly I wasn't. I would never purposely try to hurt...."

"It's okay Steffi," I interrupted. "I'm sure I must have said some horrible things to you as well."

"But you're the one who got hurt."

"Don't be so hard on yourself sis. Accidents happen right? Especially to clumsy people like me. Hey, remember the time I got those big dog slippers for Christmas, tripped over their ears and fell down the stairs almost squashing our live dog?"

"Yes, and when you landed on him, Tippy barked and barked so loud, and then started attacking the slippers as if they had first attacked you."

"And every time he saw those slippers after that, Tippy always barked and tore at the ears."

"That stupid dog was always chasing you every time you wore them."

"Yep, and I was always falling down the stairs remember?" I squeezed Steffanni's hand.

"So you'll forgive me then? You don't hate me?"

"Oh please. Of course I don't hate you. You're my little sister, my best friend, right?"

"Right," she said leaning over embracing me in a half hug. "And I always will be. Regardless of anything Melinda ever says, whether it be true or not," she whispered to me.

While we were still alone, Steffanni filled me in on the details of everything that had happened. Apparently, the pain I was feeling in my chest was due to the fact I had bruised three ribs during my tumble down the stairs, and I had also sprained my left arm. I don't know how I couldn't have noticed before she brought it to my attention, but my arm was wrapped tightly in white stretch gauze from my wrist to my elbow. Also, there was a clear plastic tube taped up my arm, running from the back of my left hand to a bag of fluids that hung above my bed. Before Steffanni could say anything further, mom and Nurse Campbell both entered the room followed by a tall, slender man, with short blonde hair, thick red rimmed glasses, and a tight lipped smile.

"Hello Jenniffer, my name is Dr. Keyes," the man introduced himself. "It's good to see you so alert and vocal." I watched him warily as he picked up a clipboard from somewhere at the foot of my bed, and flipped pages back and forth. He looked at his watch, scribbled something quickly, put the clipboard down, and moved to stand beside me. "So how is our patient feeling?" He asked.

"It hurts to talk," I said insecurely. "Or if I breathe in too deeply."

"Well that is expected of someone with injuries and conditions such as yours. A nurse will bring you something to ease your discomfort soon. Now then, can you sit up for me please Jenniffer."

Still unsure whether or not to trust him, I decided it was probably in my best interest for the time being to just co-operate and do as he asked. At least until I had my bearings. I sat up slowly as far as I could using my right arm as support. Repeatedly he pressed a cold stethoscope on my bare back, my chest, then my back again. He took my blood pressure while sitting up, and then again after I had laid back down. The pressure was so tight when the cuff was inflated, that it felt like my good arm was going to break before the tension finally released. He looked to Nurse Campbell with what seemed an unsatisfied, tenebrous expression, and repeated the entire procedure a second time.

"Ninety six over fifty one," he stated removing the cuff again. He shone a small bright light into both my eyes, clicking it on and off like a ball point pen, and then clipped it over his white smock pocket. "Do you mind if I ask you a few questions now Jenniffer? Mainly generalities we need for patient records. Nothing too personal I assure you."

"I guess not," I said. "What is it you want to know?"

"Great. First off then, do you know how tall you are?"

"An inch or so over five feet."

"So what would you say? About five foot two then?"

"Around there."

"And how much do you weigh?"

I didn't answer. *Why did he need to know how fat I was? So much for no personal questions,* I thought. This was none of his business.

"You don't know what your weight is Jenniffer? Or is it that you don't want to tell me?"

I shook my head no, and looked down.

"Get her on the scale as soon as she gets up to use the facilities," Dr. Keyes said, turning to Nurse Campbell who nodded. Then his attention was back to me. "What is the date of your last menstrual cycle?"

What? Again I didn't answer. Now he had really gone too far. That was definitely none of his damned business. Nobody's business but my own, and for that matter, his direct dry tone was starting to make me angry. This doctor was completely untrustworthy in my newly formed opinion, and I wasn't going to let him trick me into telling him anything else. Also, if he thought for one minute that he was going to get Nurse Campbell or anyone else to weigh me, he had another thing coming.

"Okay Jenniffer. We can leave things at that for tonight. I'll come back and see you in the morning after I've had a chance to review all your test results. We can talk more then about your condition and treatment options available to you for the duration of your stay."

I looked over at Mom and Steffanni for some understanding as Doctor Keyes spoke quietly with Nurse Campbell by the door, giving us all a quick nod and smile before exiting the room. *What exactly did he mean by my condition I wanted to know. More-so, what did he mean by the duration of my stay? Just how long did they plan on keeping me in here anyway?*

"Mom," I spoke out as loudly as I could. "I want to go home!"

"You are in no shape to be going anywhere my dear girl," said Nurse Campbell who was now fiddling with the tubing at the back of my hand. "No need to worry and get yourself all worked up now either. You are in the best of hands here, and we'll take such good care of you, you'll be home and back to your old self in what will feel like no time at all."

Don't worry? I wanted to scream so loud at all of them. *Didn't anyone get it at all? Getting back to my old self was what I didn't want. That was exactly what I was afraid of. They were all going to make me fatter again!*

Another nurse entered the room carrying a tray, and gave Nurse Campbell a hypodermic needle filled with a small amount of clear fluid, and then left the room just as quickly. I watched as Nurse Campbell fidgeted.

"What is that?" I asked.

"This is an intravenous tube," she said while writing on the bag that hung on the stainless steel pole above me. "And this is the saline solution we are administering to you through it."

"Why do I have it?" I asked. "What is it going to do to me?" I panicked.

"Nothing to worry about dear. It's a simple solution of distilled water, salt and sugar mostly. Basically it is like a sports drink that will help to re-hydrate and nourish your system."

No, no, no! The voice in my head screamed. *They can't do this. Don't let them do this!* She turned over my arm reading my name on the plastic band clipped around my wrist, and picked up the needle brought by the other nurse.

"Everything that goes through this tubing flows directly into your bloodstream providing the quickest results. This is some pain medication I'm giving you now," she said injecting the fluid from the needle directly into the tube taped down to my wrist. "You should be feeling better shortly, and will most likely sleep through most of the night." She tucked a small white box attached to another wire, with a yellow button, under my hip. "If you have to get up to use the bathroom, or need anything at all, just press that button and a buzzer will sound at the nurses' station at the other end of the hall. I'll be back to check on you later otherwise."

Trying hopelessly to fight the overwhelming grogginess I was suddenly feeling, I listened to Mom and Steffanni talking to me for what only seemed a couple of seconds before they were all of a sudden exiting the room. Leaving me all alone.

"Wait!" I heard myself scream out. "How many calories and fat grams do you think were in that needle and this intravenous stuff?" I mumbled. I didn't hear either a response, or the closing of the door before my eyes did. I was suddenly asleep.

13

After saying their goodbyes for the night, Victoria and Steffanni passed Dr. Keyes in the hallway when walking past the nursing station.

"Mrs. Klark," he called out. "If I may have a few minutes of your time before you leave this evening, I think it would be in your daughter's best interest."

"Forgive me, please. You are Doctor?"

"Keyes. Dr. Thomas Keyes."

"Yes, of course. How can I help you?" The seriousness in his face caused Victoria to take hold of her younger daughter's hand in a tight grip. "Everything is going to be okay with Jenniffer isn't it? You have told us everything, haven't you?"

He motioned with his hand to a vacant bench a few steps down the hall, where they all moved to and sat down.

"I hope you don't take offense to me being candid with you here, but despite what either of your daughters may have told you or your husband, I do not believe that Jenniffer falling down that flight of stairs was just an accident. Not any more than I believe her extremely low weight and frailty is the result of a lasting virus or flu."

"I don't understand. What exactly is it you are suggesting Doctor? That one of or both my daughter's are liars?"

"Forgive me but yes, objectively speaking I am. Look," he said. "Although I won't have anything concrete to base my diagnosis on until I have all of Jenniffer's lab results back, I firmly believe that your daughter is suffering from an eating disorder." He paused seeing the eyes looking back to him filling with fear, sadness, and denial. "I'm sorry Mrs. Klark. I know none of this can be easy for you to hear, but unfortunately in your daughters case...."

"Stop there, wait .... a what?" Victoria interrupted. "An eating disorder?" Victoria felt Steffanni tighten the grip on her hand, but didn't turn her head. She maintained her direct eye contact with Dr. Keyes sensing a sincerity and deep concern in his eyes. "No, you're putting us on. An eating disorder? Well that is absolutely ridiculous." She paused, then rambled on. "Not my Jenni. She is too smart for any such a thing. You have to be wrong. This is all just some kind of joke right?"

Dr. Keyes slowly shook his head.

"I wish I could tell you it was Mrs. Klark, but I assure you, this definitely is no joking matter. This is actually all very serious." His voice softened to more of a confidant and friend than that of a physician. "In Jenniffer's case," he continued, "it is a condition known medically as anorexia nervosa. She is showing signs of bulimia as well, which makes this an even more dangerous mix. From the looks of things, I don't suspect Jenniffer has been suffering for years as some cases I've seen, but in the few months I believe she has been suffering, she has been extremely demanding of her body."

"You speak as though your diagnosis is already conclusive without having to see any of Jenniffer's lab work?"

"I believe it is. Yes."

"But I thought this anorexia, eating disorder, or whatever you call it, is something that is associated with teenage girls and celebrities. Something they get or have .... not something for grown up, twenty eight year old women?"

"Well yes, typically eating disorders are made public by the media, and are generally associated to those groups. Realistically though, eating disorders are not in any way defined by gender, age, race or social status."

"Ok, so if you are right, and I am not agreeing that you are, how do we fix it? If this is what Jenniffer has, how do we make her better?"

"Mrs. Klark, anorexia is not something that is caught like the chicken pox or the common cold, and it definitely isn't something that can be fixed, or cured overnight as timely as such. Anorexia, as with all self harming psychosis is a behaviour that develops and progresses over a lengthy period of time. It can take twice the amount of time to reverse these destructive patterns and allow the body to heal itself. In your daughter's case, getting her to realize and admit that she even has a problem is going to be the first crucial step towards recovery. I'm afraid that in itself could prove more difficult than you may think. Even if Jenniffer is willing to admit she has an eating disorder, she may not be willing to let go of it. You have to be prepared that she may not want to get better."

"That's nonsense. Why wouldn't she want to get better?"

"I know this is hard to wrap your head around, but for some patients their eating disorder is a comfort to them, like a best friend if you will. It is such a big part of who they are and how they manage their life, it becomes their whole identity. They don't know who they are without it, and therefore are terrified to live without it. Even if they want to, they can't let it go."

"Wonderful," Victoria said in a hushed voice. "My daughter comes into the hospital to be assessed for a fall down some stairs in my house, and leaves crazy with some mental illness."

"Why do you think my sister has an eating disorder?" Steffanni spoke up.

"I have unfortunately seen quite a few girls, young women, even males throughout the years who have suffered with anorexia, and or bulimia. Frankly, it is quite upsetting when I think of just how many patients I have seen come in and out of this hospital alone, besides my private practice. Your sister Jenniffer, she exhibits many of the symptoms associated with these disorders."

"Like what?" Asked Steffanni.

"Many of the symptoms you may have noticed yourselves, but passed them off as symptomatic of the flu she has been telling you she has. Others you wouldn't question. Because Jenniffer lives on her own she can conceal things quite easily from you as well."

"Okay, so things like what though?" Steffanni prompted blatantly.

"Things like whether or not she has been eating regularly or exercising excessively for starters. Just looking at Jenniffer, even before doing a routine examination, I can see that she is extremely dehydrated. Her skin is grey, her eyes are deeply sunken, and her hair is brittle as straw."

"She gave herself a bad home permanent," Victoria mumbled in a heavy-hearted low voice.

"Also, the back of her throat is red and irritated," continued Dr. Keyes. "Her glands are inflamed, her teeth are showing rapidly increased signs of unnatural decay, and she has numerous scars and scabbed scratch marks on the backs of her knuckles and both her hands. These are all indicators that she has been self inducing vomiting."

"My sister-in-law said she thought Jenniffer was doing that. She told us she even caught Jenni doing that a couple weeks ago."

"Is there anything else?" Asked Victoria.

"Her blood pressure is very low, and she is showing signs of arrhythmia which concerns me. I've ordered an EKG and her to be monitored until tomorrow morning. My guess too by her apparent low weight, is that her body has quit menstruating, which is why she refused to answer me. She is probably suffering from early onset osteoporosis, which is why she cracked ribs in her short fall, anaemia which explains her low energy levels you disclosed, and a dangerous electrolyte imbalance. This would be mostly due to the vomiting, but I suspect she has been abusing diet pills, diuretics, laxatives, and anything else she could get her hands on to increase weight loss as well. I'll know more once I have gone over her lab work. I'd also like to schedule her for an ultrasound, GI endoscopy, and a few other tests if she would be willing, but I haven't come across an anorexic or bulimic yet, who has agreed to any of these procedures co-operatively."

"I just don't understand any of this!" Sighed Victoria. "It is all so hard to believe, yet even try to understand. I know .... our entire family knows," she continued, looking to Steffanni for support, "that Jenniffer has been ill with something for quite some time now, but this? As her mother, don't you think I would know if my oldest daughter was involved in something so appalling? If she was deliberately hurting herself?"

"And you are not alone in that thinking either Mrs. Klark. Let me assure you, it is quite natural to feel that way when faced with the realization that a child, or any loved one is partaking in a self destructing, self harming behaviour. It is never easy to see someone you love in harms way, yet even more difficult when they are the person deliberately putting themselves there. It is especially difficult in circumstances like your families' where Jenniffer lives apart from you. You don't see her day to day adversity, but are forced to take a back seat and helplessly accept her choices. In this case ...."

"Enough!" Victoria exploded rising to her feet. "Look Dr. Keyes, I appreciate your concern here, and I applaud also your devotion to patient care. However, I will not believe that this type of monster you describe is my daughter. I just can't! I cannot believe that she has done any of these things purposely, only to look me directly in the face and lie to me about it. I have to stand by what my daughter tells me as truth, and that all this is simply nothing more than a bad run in with the flu. I'm sorry. Now if you will excuse us, we have to go." Victoria grabbed Steffanni's arm in one hand and extended the other to Dr. Keyes. "If you would be so kind, please let Jenniffer know when she wakes that I will return first thing in the morning to see her."

"Gladly," he said, firmly shaking her hand. "If you will do something for me also. Just give what we have discussed some thought. Don't shrug things off too quickly is all I ask. I hate to say it, but your daughters' life may depend on it." Victoria pulled her hand away agitated by his resolute insistence. "There are some excellent books on the subject of eating disorders in the hospitals library located on the fifth floor. On your way out, I urge you to stop in and sign a couple of them out. You can give my name as the referring physician."

"If there is any change in Jenniffer's condition throughout the night, or she wakes and needs me, will you please have someone call me if not herself?" Victoria asked.

"Definitely."

Steffanni didn't speak a word to her mother as she watched the elevator door close slowly in front of them, or when it opened again to let them out in the main lobby. She didn't speak a word either when her mother stepped back again and then pushed the elevator button for the fifth floor. A sobering silence remained between them for the next hour until after they were home. Before getting out of the car Victoria passed Steffanni a bag containing three books she had signed out from the hospitals library, and asked her to keep them until she had spoken with her father. All Steffanni said to her mother then, was thank you.

14

The next couple of days for me was the beginning of sheer hell on earth, and the battles I fought with my family and numerous medical practitioners spun me in round-the-clock circles like a spider spinning an endless web. The arguments with my mother were however the worst, and pretty much always the same.

"Jenni, you don't sound well. Do you want me to go in and visit you for awhile? We could play cards or something."

"No mom. I'm fine. Besides, I'm leaving this place first thing tomorrow morning."

"Oh Jenni, this again? Please tell me you're not."

"I am."

"But honey, you need to be in a hospital. You need to be in a doctor's care."

"No, I don't! And I'm not staying here in this hospital one more day!"

"It's only been three days since your fall and you still need more rest and nourishment to gain back your strength and to get healthy again. Quite frankly Jenni, the doctors are not the only ones who are worried about your weight and constant refusal to treatment. Your father and I are sick to death with worry, and your poor sister, well she is just terrified that you are going to be too ill even to attend her wedding, let alone stand up with her."

"I'm sorry you all feel that way mom, but I have been here long enough, and this is all getting to be quite exaggerated. I'm not trying to upset you, but I am not staying here after tonight. I just can't and that's that!"

"Well if you won't stay in there, how about transferring to a different hospital for awhile? Or what about one of those other treatment centres that Dr. Keyes suggested? Like the places that specialize in eating disorders where they can really help you with all of this and you can get better?"

"Mom, why won't you believe me? I do not have an eating disorder okay! I am not going into any other hospital, and I'm not going into any treatment centre anywhere else either."

"Couldn't you at least give it some more thought Jenni?"

"No, I won't! Mom, you are not listening! I said, I don't need any help!"

"But honey, you do, and your father and I both agree with your doctors that you need to stay in treatment. You need to stay in the hospital long enough to gain some of your strength back, and you need professionals to help to deal with all of this Jenni."

"Oh for the love of God Mother! For the last time, there is nothing wrong with me! Why can't you all understand that? I don't need to be treated for anything, and I don't need any professional's help! What I do need in fact is to be left alone!"

"So what? That's it then? You just expect all of us, everyone who loves you to just do nothing but sit around and watch you self destruct?"

"I am not self destructing." I said more solemnly.

"You most certainly are. You are slowly wasting away."

"Mom, stop. Come on, please don't start crying on me again?"

"Stop crying Jenniffer? How am I to stop crying when my oldest daughter is slowly killing herself?"

"Stop being so overly mellow dramatic will you mother. I am not killing myself."

"But you are Jenni. By slowly starving yourself to death, you are."

"I am not starving."

"You haven't eaten for days I bet."

"I eat all the time."

"What then? Tell me what have you eaten?"

I paused trying to remember what it was and when the last time I actually ate by choice had been. I couldn't.

"Well they are pumping me full of all this intravenous garbage in here you know, so I haven't actually been hungry. But I have eaten some things."

"Exactly! And that right there is the point! You haven't listened to a single word Dr. Keyes or any of the others have said to you over the last forty-eight hours have you? You can't just survive on water alone Jenniffer! Your body is starving and you are dying because you are not eating enough. You need to eat!"

"Whatever mom." I sighed heavily. "What do those high priced doctors know anyhow?"

"They know that you are incapable of taking proper care of yourself right now."

"Well I say, I have been taking care of myself for years on my own until now, and I think I have done quite well I might add."

"Until recently, yes you have. But lately you haven't and your father and I tend to agree with your doctors that for now you need to stay in a hospital."

"And I don't. I'm an adult now mom and you can tell me anything you want, but what you can't do, is send me to my room anymore because you don't agree with things I've done or am going to do. I make my own decisions now. I'm not a child anymore."

"Well you will always be my child Jenni. Look, if you absolutely refuse to be in treatment somewhere, will you at least come back here and stay with us for awhile again? I know your dad would like that, and Steffi would too. If nothing more, you can at least give me some comfort in knowing that you are not alone if something does happen or if you need something."

"You mean close by you so that you can all spy on me."

"No, I mean close by so I can help you get through all this."

"I'm not going to eat everything you put on the table in front of me and get fatter again, just so that you can all be happy and go jumping up and down like you just won some stupid prize at the carnival if that is what you think."

"This isn't a game Jenni, and no-one is trying to or going to make you fat. Just healthy."

"Whatever."

"No, not whatever. So?

"So what?"

"Will you come home?"

"Fine mom, I will go to your place. But I'll eat what I want, when I want, and only how much I want. I will go home to my own apartment if you push me. Understand?"

"So you will come home then?"

"If that's what it takes to get you to stop crying, and get off my back. I will for awhile just to prove to you that I don't need to be in some crazy treatment centre for something I do not have, and you can see for yourself that I am fine okay."

"Okay then. Do you want me to pick you up now?"

"No, it's late now and I'm exhausted. I'm going to go back to sleep. Picking me up tomorrow morning will be fine."

"I am going to go make some tea and tell your father what we've discussed, and let him know what we've agreed upon. Your sister too. She will be happy."

"Just know that I am signing myself out of this place right after breakfast is served in the morning which is at is eight o'clock. After that I will be gone."

"Fine Jenniffer, if that is what you want. Just promise me you won't leave before we get there to pick you up. There may be traffic, and you know your dad likes to drive slow."

"I'll wait for you."

"Promise me you won't leave before we get there?"

"I promise, okay! I promise!"

"All right then. I'll go talk to your father now, and you go get some rest."

"You can stop crying now too mom, and I'll see you first thing in the morning. I am hanging up now okay? Good night."

"Sleep well then. Oh, and Jenni .... I love you."

"I love you too Mom. Good night."

15

Stuart sat motionless behind his desk in his den with his elbows firmly pressed over an array of papers, and his palms supporting his slumped head. He was known to sit like this only when something was very wrong. When he didn't know what he could do to make the slightest positive difference in a bad situation, and he faced something he could not fix. The usual culprit was his work. A guilty client looking to be pardoned, or an innocent man facing a lengthy sentence term. The case at hand this time however was a personal one, and the decision needed to be made was tearing him in more than one direction from inside and out in all directions. He felt himself losing before the trial, and he was out of his element determining the case at hand. He was going to have to be his own judge and jury of one in this circumstance and he felt numb; deadlocked with no reprieve.

"Stuart," Victoria spoke quietly, entering the den. "We need to talk."

"About?"

"About Jenni," she said closing the door tightly behind her. "Stu, I am more worried about her now. More than ever. I don't think she is getting any better." Victoria stared across to her husband. "I actually think she may be getting worse!"

Stuart stood up and walked over to the window, and stared outside for a long time. He watched two robins relentlessly plunge their beaks into the rain soaked lawn under their feet in their own quest for food.

"I just don't understand it," he said. "Why the hell won't she just eat? Eat something? Anything? People don't just not eat Victoria, and I'm sorry, she may be our daughter, and I love her, but rational people don't go and throw up everything afterward when they have eaten either! It all seems so much nonsense to me Vic, all this talk of hers about being fat. For Christ's sake, she must weigh what now, the same as she did when she was twelve?"

"On her admission papers the other day, I read that she weighed eighty seven pounds."

Stuart turned to face his wife seeing the same desperation in her eyes he was wrestling within himself.

"Have I not been a good father? Have I not provided her with enough over the years? Too much? Was I not there for her enough as a child? What is it?" He cried. "Is this the prolonged result of some overblown middle child syndrome? Does she not feel that I love her enough? For God's sake Victoria, does she not know that it's because I love her so much that I'm so distraught? Does she expect us to just sit back and watch her continue this destructive behaviour forever? Wait for her to die?" Stuart took his wife in his arms and held her tightly, letting out a heavy sigh.

"Every day is like a nightmare for me too you know." Victoria sobbed. "The same horror plays every minute of the day while I'm awake, and I am constantly searching for some sense of normalcy in all of this. When I can sleep, my dreams are all consuming of the same. My heart aches so deeply for this nightmare to end, yet I am so scared that its end will be the end of Jenniffer also. I don't know what's worse anymore, staying awake worrying the end will come, or waking, fearing that while I slept it has. Stuart I can't lose her!" Victoria cried out trembling. "She's our oldest daughter. We can't let her die. Stu, please, don't let me lose her!"

Stuart held his wife a little tighter, then pulled away and wiped her eyes.

"She is signing herself out of the hospital in the morning. She absolutely refuses to stay there any longer." Victoria sniffled. "She refuses to listen to reason."

"So she is going back home, where she will be all by herself to do or not do whatever she wants?"

"Not exactly. She has actually agreed to come to our home here. I told her we would pick her up at eight, but.... well I don't think ....."

"I know. You're going to say you don't think she will stay very long here either before going back to her own place."

"Stu, honestly. We can't let her."

Stuart sat back down behind his desk and pulled open the top drawer lifting out a manilla envelope given to them by Dr. Keyes.

"She will hate me you know?" He said. "She will hate us both."
"I know."
"She will fight everyone involved every step of the way."
"Yes she will."

Stuart dumped the contents of the envelope out onto his desk. A brochure for Caitlynne's Place - Home and Treatment Centre for Victims of Eating Disorders, a business card, and a pre-filled admissions package.

"Are you sure this is the right thing for us to do here?"

"Honestly Stu, I don't know if it is or it isn't, but Jenniffer isn't going to get any help on her own and we've already tried everything else." Victoria took a pen from its holder and held it out to her husband. "What I do know for sure though, is that I'd rather have our daughter alive and hating us than the alternative. I don't see how we have any other choice left now. Do you?"

Stuart took the pen, signed the papers and slid both back across to his wife who then signed her name alongside his. Next he made two short telephone calls. One to Caitlynne's Place and the second to the courthouse, after which he took both his wife's hands firmly in his.

"Judge Raemous is going to meet us in his chambers at seven tomorrow morning, and everything will be in place when we pick up Jenni at eight. We can sign her in to Caitlynne's Place anytime after ten. Admissions said if we fax a copy of the court order along with her forms prior to our arrival, it will make things a lot smoother for all involved when we get her there. They suggest we pick her up at the hospital and say we are going for a Saturday morning drive to fill in time. I'll make up some excuse about having to go out of town to drop off papers to a client, and a nice day for a drive. She will believe that. It's misleading I know, but it may be the only way to get her there."

"And they'll take care of her, and keep her safe there right?"

"And make sure she stays alive."

16

"This is an outrage!" I screamed at my parents. "You can't do this to me! You can't!"

My mom stretched out her hand to my arm trying to console me.

"Don't touch me!" I growled twisting away.

"Honey please. Try to understand your father's and my position. We felt we had no other choice. We knew you wouldn't come on your own, and you're not getting any better at home."

I glared at my mother with sheer discontent; then at my father.

"And you. You lied to me! How could you lie to me Daddy? You said you had to drop something off for work somewhere, that it would be nice to have company along for the ride. What you really meant was to drop off the problem which is me, right? Well go ahead! Dump me off on someone else's doorstep with your flashy court papers and leave me behind with strangers! How could you? You've been constantly condemning me for lying and breaking trust for weeks, and then you yourself go and lie to me? I guess I'm supposed to take it though, 'cause you're the parent and I'm the lowly, or rather, abandoned child now right?"

A tall, evenly tanned lady with shimmering, shoulder length, summer blonde hair, and a brilliant white smile approached us, while another man and woman stood a few feet behind.

"Hello Jenniffer. I'm Catherine Shaw," she said cheerfully extending her hand toward me.

I rejected her hand. I didn't want to be rude or impolite, but I didn't want to be here either. She smiled then shook my parents' hands.

"She likes to be called Jenni," my mother stated.

"What the hell do you know?" I snapped sarcastically.

Catherine nodded to my parents, then turned to me.

"Okay Jenniffer. Why don't you say your goodbyes, and then we'll go and get you settled in."

I kept my body stiff as a board while my mother hugged me, and whispered shakily in my ear that she loved me. Then my dad hugged me.

"It will be okay honey," he said. "They are going to take good care of you here, and you will get better."

I couldn't fight the tears anymore. They streamed over my cheeks like tiny waterfalls and dripped from my chin. Dad hugged me tighter for a minute, kissed my forehead, and then stepped away.

"Honestly honey, it will all be okay. You'll see."

"Daddy please?" I pleaded with him one last time. "Don't leave me here. I will do whatever you want me to Daddy. I promise! I will eat anything you want me to, anything you say, if you just take me home. Please Daddy, I'll be good, I promise. I don't belong here!"

Stuart took his wife by the hand, nodded to Catherine and turned away. For the moment I felt numb as I watched my mom and dad both turn their backs to me and I was led in the opposite direction toward the front door. It was really happening. They were really leaving me behind.

"Jenniffer, it's time to go get settled in now. Your parents can come back and visit you again soon."

"Don't bother!" I screamed to their backs. "I never want to see either one of you again! Do you hear me? I hate you for betraying me like this! I hate you! I hate you both!"

My parents never looked back. They just left me standing there in a strange place, with a crowd of strangers. Twenty eight years old, and I was stripped of all my rights. My life was in no way my own any longer. What I had yet to realize, was that it hadn't been for a very many weeks already.

Catherine bent down to pick up the suitcase my parents had pre-packed for me and hidden in the trunk of the car.

"I can carry my own belongings thank you," I said, reaching past her, grabbing the handle.

"Very well then," Catherine said smiling. "I'll show you to your room and give you some time to settle in before orientation and dinner."

I followed her down a narrow hallway, up a winding staircase, to an open space surrounded by closed rooms with numbers and nameplates on each rooms door. Stopping at a door with the number two, one empty name frame, and one that said 'Ameliah', and knocked. Not hearing a reply, Catherine opened the door, and peered in before opening it all the way.

"It looks as if your roommate is out," she said. "But I'm sure she won't be too long. She was very happy to hear she was going to have some company for awhile. We try to room people together that we think are good matches, and from what your parents have told me, I think the two of you will get along very well."

I didn't say anything as she spoke, but rather stood in the doorway trying desperately not to convey on my face my curiosity as to what my parents had indeed told her, or the excruciating pain in my upper body and limbs from carrying my own bag.

"Well, as you can see that is your side of the room," she said pointing to barren shelves and an empty closet to the left. The dresser and the desk are both yours to store your things in, and you share the washroom. Any questions?"

I shook my head.

"I know this is hard for you now, but know that everyone here is struggling with the same demons you are in one way or another. Everyone here is fighting the same disordered eating battles." Catherine took my suitcase out of my clutches, walked across the room and set it on what was now going to be my bed. "My husband and our staff are all here because we care Jenniffer, and we all want to help you win your battle. We're all on the same side, even though it may not feel that way for you now."

She went to the window, and drew back the heavy, olive green drape that fell to the floor, and then walked back to me at the door.

"Your roommates name is Ameliah, as it says on the door, and unless you prefer to be known here by a different nickname, I will introduce you as Jenniffer, and make your nameplate the same." She paused, as if waiting for my clarification, but I just stood there. "Okay then, so Jenniffer, it is two o'clock now and I will come back at three to give you a tour of the rest of the house and grounds. That leaves you with about an hour to get unpacked and settled in beforehand. Still no questions?"

I didn't move.

"Well if you think of any, write them down. You will find a pen and paper in the desk and we can go over them at three. I'll see you then."

I looked at my watch when she shut the door behind me, then stood there for another fourteen minutes after I heard her last footstep in the hall disappear before I moved. *This wasn't really happening to me was it?* I questioned to myself. *My parents wouldn't really do this to me, would they? It had to be some kind of well planned out joke.* I searched the room with my eyes, not moving my head. There had to be a hidden candid camera somewhere I couldn't see. I turned quickly and jerked open the heavy room door, truly half expecting to see mom and dad laughing wildly in the foyer with all the other pranksters they had involved. There wasn't a person in sight; only silence. I quietly pushed the door shut again and retreated to the bed on the side of the room shown to be mine.

I was twenty eight years old and living in a country where I was declared an adult, paid taxes, and free to choose my own path. I was old enough to vote, to drink, to smoke, to drive, and to live on my own independently which is exactly where I should be now. Instead, I was stuck here in a strange place, locked up like a wild animal, trapped and caged with all my rights and freedoms taken from me.

17

Caitlynne's Place is a forty five minute drive North of Edson, in the Pineridge Valley, owned and operated by Dr. Brian Shaw and his wife Dr. Catherine Shaw, a registered dietician. Originally their private residence, after losing their only daughter to anorexia nervosa, Catherine and Brian, decided to convert their forty eight hundred square foot home into an eating disorder treatment lodge. It took almost two years to complete the renovations, and in 1996 they opened the doors to Caitlynne's Place in their daughter's honour, with hopes of helping other sufferers win their battles in their wars with eating disorders. Within three weeks of opening the doors, all sixteen beds upstairs were filled, and there was a waiting list with nine additional names of other families looking for new treatment options and hope. Brian and Catherine very much viewed eating disorders as a round-the-clock double edged sword, and all sufferers victims. During the first eight years Caitlynne's Place had been open, it housed a total of just over four hundred victims. Six of them who sadly fell prey to their disease, and lost their battle to death.

At precisely three o'clock, just as she said she would, Catherine Shaw returned to take me on my orientation tour of the house and grounds. As much as I hated being here, I decided for the time being, it would be best if I just did what Catherine wanted me to, and familiarize myself with my new surroundings. As we walked through and around the house I didn't speak a word. I nodded whenever Catherine asked me if I understood something she was showing or telling me, and I followed silently behind her like an obedient dog on a leash.

Caitlynne's Place was by far the largest house I had ever been in, and really by all means, it was a resort.

On the lower level of the house, there was a common area with a complete home theatre system, and a vast collection of movies. Adjoining, there was a large sunken area with four computer desks, all internet ready, three walls cased with books, and a quiet sitting area around a wood burning fireplace like you'd find in the back of a chalet. The common rooms were open to all guests with privileges throughout the day and night, and apparently privileges were something earned and determined by cooperating in the program I would find more out about later. Other rooms on the main floor such as the kitchen, pantry, dining, laundry, utility, and recreation, were only for specified uses, at specified times. Two of the areas completely restricted were the Shaws' chambers, and the living quarters for Amy Larson, the Recreational Director. At the front of the house where I had come in at reception, there was an additional set of bathrooms, and down the hall from there was an examining room, and two separate office spaces. One door had a name plate imprinted with 'Dr. Brian Shaw', and the other 'Dr. S. Burman'. I would later find out that Dr. Burman is a visiting psychologist that travels in daily for appointments Mondays to Fridays. At the back of the house, Catherine led me down a set of stairs to another lower basement level where it separated into two areas. The front contained rows of floor to ceiling filing cabinets, and wall to wall shelves of supplies for the home. The back half was closed off behind locked doors, where Paul and Patricia Saunders resided. Paul is the house Chef, and his wife Patricia is a registered accountant who also helps with administrations.

The properties' grounds outside were just as overwhelming. I followed Catherine through manicured gardens planted with many diversified flowers and grasses, as she led me down a cobblestone path that meandered from the main front entrance of the house, around to the back where it circled a beautiful cascading fountain then disappeared beyond a tree-line. There, three different paths branched off into the sparsely forested acreage, all looping back to the central fountain. One path circled around a large fruit and vegetable garden, another around an extensive herb garden, and the other led to a small shallow pond with a massive old willow tree shading half of it, and a small waterfall trickling at the opposite end.

Although I had many questions when Catherine and I returned to my room, only one seemed of any relevance.

"When can I go home?" I asked.

"When you are better," she replied with a smile. "And not before then."

18

While I had been out, a new name plate with my name in bold print had replaced the empty slot on the door, and the girl occupying the other side of the room had also returned.

I smiled and walked sheepishly past her going directly into the bathroom without saying anything. After I closed the door, I noticed there wasn't any way to lock it from the inside. I reopened it and looked above the outer handle. There was a key bolt lock on the outside, but no lock for the inside. I quickly washed my face and hands, and then hurried back to my side of the room.

"This is your first time in a treatment facility isn't it?"

"Yep, sure is." I sighed heavily, and sat down on my bed, looking out the window opposite her direction.

"Well trust me. If you have to be in somewhere, you want to be in here. This is a five star luxury resort compared to most of them. The place I was before this was like a prison compared to here. Sandpaper bed sheets at night, and stale oatmeal for breakfast each day. And the staff, no comparison whatsoever. They're angels here compared to the wardens at most other places. So your name is Jenniffer right?" I made no reply, but the girl continued to introduce herself regardless. "I'm Ameliah. Ameliah Prescott. They probably told you that when they brought you into the room earlier though, right? And it also says so on the door. That is how I know your name too."

I flopped down over my bed and closed my eyes.

"It's all okay. Trust me, I understand and won't take it personally if you don't want to talk right now. I wasn't really in the mood to make friends with anyone the first time they locked me up in a strange place. Nobody else ever does either, if that's of any comfort to you knowing. We can always talk later."

I didn't have the energy to talk. I just couldn't find it in me to even try at that point. I was physically and mentally played out and exhausted. *Why was all this happening to me? And why was this girl who didn't even know me at all, whom I had just met, being so nice to me when I was being so ignorant and rude to her?*

"Hey, hey you over there," Ameliah's voice broke into my sleep awhile later. "Are you coming or not?"

"What?" I asked forcing open my eyes. "Coming? Going where?"

"The dining room. It's a quarter to five. Didn't you hear the bell?"

"No," I yawned. "Sorry, I must have fallen asleep."

"Well I'm going down now. I just got my pass privileges back yesterday, and I don't want to jeopardize them by being late. Do you remember where the dining room is?"

I nodded apethetically and watched her leave. Then I went back to sleep.

When I awoke again, it was well after dark. The only light was from a small desk lamp on Amelaih's side of the room where she was reading, and I couldn't help but stare. Long chestnut hair framed her thin oval face well defined by her high cheekbones and light skin tone. She had deep set, dark brown eyes and a dazzling white smile that would put a Cheshire cat to shame. She was sitting at her desk in perfect posture which showed off her slender torso, and although I couldn't see all of her legs, there was definitely no sign of flab spreading anywhere over the chair she was sitting on. She was nothing like me. She was beautiful. She was thin. And *maybe, just maybe*, I thought to myself now fully awake, *she could teach me how to be thin too.*

"Excuse me?" I cleared my throat. "Um excuse me, Ameliah?" She glanced over smiling.

"Sorry for interrupting you. I just wanted to apologize for being so rude to you earlier."

"Don't sweat it. And you're not interrupting me by any means. More like saving me from this boring magazine my dad sent me."

"What is it you're reading?"

"Aviator's monthly," she said showing me the cover.

"Ahh, that does sound exciting." I sat up and rubbed my legs trying to get the circulation going. "I'm Jenniffer by the way." I said getting to my feet, crossing the room to shake her hand.

"Nice to meet you." She said accepting my hand.

I pulled myself up and sat cross legged on the foot of her bed.

"Am I going to be in trouble for missing dinner earlier, and not going downstairs? I asked her unknowingly.

"Nah, don't worry too much about it. The new girls always get away with ignoring their first days' snacks and meals. It's pretty much the same as everywhere, but be prepared, you might be able to get away with it again tomorrow, but come Monday it will be '*The first day of the rest of your life*' again right?"

I must have looked as baffled as I felt by her answer because she suddenly seemed a little confused too.

"Yep, I'm right, she said smiling. "This is your first time in isn't it?"

"Why do you keep asking me that?"

"Because that look of tough innocence on your face is a dead giveaway."

I looked down.

"Hey, don't worry. It's hard for everyone the first time, but you'll soon catch on. You just have to learn how to fly under their radar, and give in to what they want from you. That is, if you really do want to get out of here."

"Of course I want out of here!" I snapped. "Why would anyone want to be stuck in here?"

"Well I wouldn't go around saying this to just anybody, but some people I know would love the chance to stay here forever. There's no judgement or artificial standard to have to live up to in here, and not only that but it is a safe place to be in, even when you hate it. It's a catch twenty two. On the other hand though, some people will do whatever it takes to just get out as fast as they can so that they can have their freedom and privacy back to do whatever they choose. They're always the ones you see come and go over and over again every few months."

"Wow. You sound like you really know what you're talking about. How many times have you been here?"

"Here? At Caitlynne's Place? Once for three months last fall. I was in a Sick Kids Hospital on four different occasions, on the psych ward at my parents' local hospital too many times to count, and through a six month program at some clinic in L.A. a few years back. This will be my last stay here."

"But that's crazy. There's not a thing wrong with you. From what I can see you look great. You are so young and so beautiful."

"Careful how you use the word crazy around here," she laughed. "Some people will definitely take offense to that. As for me, the last time I saw my chart it said that I'm a 'resistant anorexic with perfectionist, obsessive compulsive, bipolar tendencies', whatever that means. What about yourself? What got you put in here?"

"I'm just fat. And no-one else wants me to diet."

"Anorexic. I thought so. You throw up all the time too, don't you?"

How the hell did she know that, I wondered.

"Yeah, you look like you have bulimic outbursts. You're probably a flusher too, right?"

"A what?"

"A flusher. You know, laxative use, diuretics, that sort of thing."

I was shocked. This girl didn't even know I existed this morning, and now she seemed to know my deepest, darkest secrets, and innermost thoughts.

"How do you know all this? Does everyone in this house know everything about everybody else's business or what?"

"Not right away, but pretty much in time everyone gets to know everything about everybody. After you've been around awhile you kind of get to know things just by looking too. My last roommate was the same as you. I can tell a lot just by your skin tone and your glands, the yellow in the whites of your eyes, that sort of thing. You're not alone here though. There are six others in the house the same as you.

"Just exactly how many people are there in here?"

"Let's see," she said, starting to count on her fingers. "There's June and Donna in room one, who are both fifteen. Susie is really chatty, and the champion backgammon player in the house right now, so if you play her, good luck. We're in room two. Susan who is thirteen, and Penny, who just turned sixteen last week, are in room three. Brian and Catherine decorated the entire lounge with balloons and streamers, and threw Penny this huge sweet sixteen birthday party. It's too bad you didn't get here last week because I think it was probably the most fun anyone has ever had in rehab," she laughed. "Susie and Penny are really buddy-buddy too so watch what you say about one in front of the other if you know what I mean. Karen who is forty nine and we all call the 'lifer' because she's so old, and been here so long is in room four with Valerie who is thirty six. Valerie is a major bulimic and extremely emotional too, so you never want to use that word 'crazy' around her, or anything like it because she will completely fly off the handle. Room five has Barbara, eighteen, and Madeline, seventeen, who are both pretty quiet and keep to themselves. Room six has Brenda, eighteen, and Allison, nineteen, and in room seven, there's Jonathan. He's the only guy here so he's got a room all to himself. He is kind of shy being the only male in the house, but once he gets to know you a bit, he'll open up. He's an encyclopaedia when it comes to movie trivia, so if you're ever looking for a good movie here to watch, he can tell you them all. And then in room eight there's Elizabeth or Lizzy who is seventeen, and Kerri who is also seventeen. Kerri just got here two weeks ago, so I don't know a lot about her yet other than she's anorexic. I think she was transferred directly from another program somewhere because she's eating pretty good already, and she's not as skinny as most people when they first come in like you are. Still, they're all the same."

Ameliah just referred to me as skinny, I thought to myself and couldn't help but relish the compliment even if I didn't believe it. At least if I was going to have to stay in this place now and share a room with a stranger, I was glad I got the room I did with Ameliah as my roommate.

"How long has Karen been here?" I asked. "She's who you call the lifer, right?"

"Karen? Yep. She's been here nine months now."

"Nine months! That's almost a year!"

"Almost."

"How long have you been here?"

"Me? Going on four months this time. I still have to gain six more pounds before I can get out."

"I can't be in here for four months!" I screamed jumping angrily to my feet. "I have a business to run!"

"You own a business?"

"No, not exactly, but I manage a small Café by the river in Edson."

"Edson? That's about an hour from here with a small airport on the outskirts right?"

"You know someone there?"

"No, but I've been there, in and out before. I'm a flight attendant."

"Wow, really? I always wondered if that was as exiting as it sounded. Getting to travel all over and getting paid to see the world."

"Well I have travelled to a lot of different countries and cities but I wouldn't consider it all that exciting. The crew doesn't really ever get much time to explore or see the places we fly in and out of. Mostly just a lot of hotels and airports."

"Did you always want to be a flight attendant?"

"Gosh no. My dad's a pilot for Long Jet Airlines and an all-out fanatic about anything aerobatic. Hence the name Ameliah, after Amelia Earhart. You know, first woman to fly the Atlantic. Really I wanted to be a nurse, but to please daddy I am a flight attendant working with his airline."

"Did you ever pursue any medical school?"

"Nope. Just a dream. I know, you're probably thinking that I am crazy right, giving up on my dreams for those of someone else. Just to please my parents."

"Not at all. I actually wanted to pursue a career in sales and advertising but never left the Café since starting there. To please my parents too, I'll probably buy the damn place. If I even have a job left there to go back to after all this that is." I sat down on Ameliah's bed again and looked around the room. "Right now that job is all I have. I've got to get out of here."

"If you're the manager I'm sure your job will be held for you. What did your boss say when you told them you were going to be away?"

"I didn't know I was going to be away! I thought I was going back!"

"Going back? So you have been away then?"

"I was off work with a flu virus for a couple weeks and then admitted into Edson Memorial for a couple of days. Nothing serious, just a little low blood pressure and dehydration from being sick. My parents picked me up this morning when I was discharged and my dad said we were going to make a 'quick little detour' so he could drop off some papers to a client before we went back to their place. Needless to say more, they unloaded me here."

"Well to hell with them girl, you're older than eighteen. Sign yourself out and go home."

"If only I could. I played that card already," I said sighing heavily turning to face Ameliah. *Why was I was finding it so easy to talk to her,* I wondered. *Maybe because she was all that I had at that moment, and I desperately needed someone. Or, maybe it was because she was the first and only person who really seemed to understand me. Maybe it was both.* "My father's a lawyer," I told her, and we both laughed half heartedly as she rolled her eyes and stretched back in her chair. "Yeah, apparently he and my mom are panicking, thinking I am making myself sick on purpose or something. So my dad went and got some judge friend of his to sign some legal document stating that I was psychologically incapable of making competent choices for myself, when it came to my own health. Apparently they think I am a danger to my own physical and mental well being. Twenty eight years old, and I have no personal rights. Go figure."

"Sucks to have parents in power doesn't it?" She sighed. "I turned twenty three myself last month, but you'd think I was only five the way my parents try to treat me as well."

"Forcing you to stay here too are they?"

"Well they don't have a court order or anything, but they've threatened to try and get one if I didn't readmit myself voluntarily. It's okay though. It keeps me away from the stresses of the skies right now, and I kind of needed a rest from it all I think. Like I said before, the people are all pretty good to us here. Once you get to know them all yourself and give them a chance, I think you'll agree too."

"Well Catherine seemed nice enough, even though I wasn't very social with her earlier today. But then, I wasn't in a very social mood either."

"Her husband Brian is really nice too. He's the GP here so you'll be seeing him for regular check ups and medical things, but that's it. He doesn't usually interact with all of us as much as Catherine and the others do."

"We have to have regular checkups?"

"You bet we do," she said getting up. "But can we talk more again later? I don't mean to be rude when this is all so new to you, but I am really beat. I think I'm going to go have a shower and call it a night. Do you mind?"

"No, of course not. I am still pretty tired too, even though I guess I slept most of the evening already." I got up and walked back over to my side of the room, then turned back and called across to her. "Hey, Ameliah. Where's the lock for the inside of the bathroom door located?"

She flung her housecoat and pajamas over her shoulder and chuckled.

"I know it might seem crazy to ask such a stupid question but..."

"Sorry roomy, I wasn't laughing at you, just your innocence. You really do have a lot to learn that's for sure. There isn't a lock for the inside Jenniffer. None of the bathroom doors anywhere in the main house or guest rooms have locks from the inside. That's how they monitor the flushers. Make sure you're not spitting back up your food."

"They watch us use the bathrooms you mean?"

"If they feel they need to they do."

"But that's an infringement on my privacy!"

"In here you have no privacy. And like I said, the only way out is by following their rules and achieving the goals they set for you." She shut the bathroom door, then reopened it and stuck her head out. "By the way, if you want to store some of your personal stuff in here, my last roommate had the bottom drawer so it's empty for your use now."

Looking around the room I realized I hadn't even opened my bag and wondered what was inside. This morning I wasn't even aware that I had needed a suitcase, and tonight here it was in front of me, puffed at the seams like an overstuffed pillowcase. I tossed the blue leather case on top of my dresser and popped open the copper clasps, hesitating to unpack anything that was stored inside. With shaking hands I flipped open the top and saw a hand written note.

My Dearest Jenni,
*   If there is anything you want or need that I haven't sent with you, please let me know and I will get it to you.*
*   Love Mom.*

I took the note, crumpled and dropped it into the trash bin. I didn't have to look any further to know there was nothing more I needed or wanted from her, so instead of looking through my suitcase any further, I shut the top and crawled into bed.

19

I didn't see or speak to anybody after I woke the next day, and spent most of it again in bed facing the wall. I was aware of someone going in and out on occasion, that I concluded must be Ameliah, but I didn't acknowledge it. After not showing up again the next day for breakfast in the dining room, Catherine, accompanied by her husband Brian, and a Dr. Leslie Burman came in to see me. They all pulled up chairs from around the room and sat around my bed where I had not moved from since climbing in.

"How are you feeling today Jenniffer?" Brian asked.

"Okay I guess," I said in a slurred voice. I had been determined when I woke that I was going to stand my ground and continue making my own choices, whether my parents had me locked up in here or not. Looking into the cold stares of the three sitting around me, I could feel what strength I had slipping away like a slow leak in an old air mattress.

"That's good to hear," he said.

"Well I'd be a lot better if I could go back home," I said trying to sound firm.

"And that is why we are all here this morning Jenniffer," Catherine stated.

I pushed myself up onto my elbows, and glanced at each of them. "I can go home?"

"Yes Jenniffer, you can," said Brian clearly.

But not until you're better," Catherine cut in. "And that is why the three of us are in here with you this morning. We have to go over the game plan so that you can start taking your first steps on your road to recovery. That is the road that will take you home Jenniffer. The only road."

Instantly, I sank back into my sheets. I could feel a raging sea of loathing and anger stirring inside me, and I closed my eyes as they started to burn. *You are twenty eight years old,* I told myself. *Do not let them manipulate and gain control of you. Do not let them break you. Do not let them see you cry.*

"Just tell me straight up please," I demanded tight lipped. "How long do I have to stay in here?"

"That depends on how hard you are willing to work. There is no definite time frame." Brian answered.

I could hear the scratch of a pencil rapidly moving across paper, and opened my eyes looking for the irritating source. It was Dr. Burman. He was a short, stout man I'd put somewhere around fifty, with silver streaked, sandy brown hair, and dark bushy eyebrows that made his eyes look like tiny lasers that could see directly through anything or anyone. I knew he could see my glare out of the corner of his eye, but he never looked up to acknowledge It. He just kept on writing.

"Okay, so what do I have to do?" I asked.

"The first thing you have to do is get your weight up a bit," said Brian. "The average weight for a grown woman of your height is one hundred twenty two pounds and your weight is a dangerously low eighty seven pounds. Our goal for you is to reach a minimum of one-ten before we can even think of letting you go home."

"That's absurd!" I yelled shaking my head frantically side to side. "Uh uh. No way. I can't. I just can't. You don't understand," I pleaded with all of them. "It's too much."

Catherine leaned in to me tenderly covering my hand with hers, and her voice softened to a gentle tone like that of a mother to a child who had just fallen and scraped her knee.

"We know the thought of gaining even an ounce itself is terrifying for you at this point Jenniffer, but I promise you, in time as you grow stronger that fear will slowly diminish."

"And we're not expecting this weight gain all at once," said Brian. "However, I would like to see a gain of at least eight to ten pounds over the next couple of weeks."

My concealed tears began to fall, and Catherine placed a large manilla folder on my bedspread in front of me.

"The information in there is for you. Enclosed you will find a copy of the court order, and your admission papers. You'll notice that your parents have both signed them, but there is also a space we would encourage you to sign also. It will show good intentions on your part in cooperation with the program and your recovery. You will also find a copy of your daily timetable, which you are required to adhere to without exception starting now, and also a list outlining the rewards and consequences with regards to your conduct thereto. It is up to you to familiarize yourself with your own schedule, and attend all your appointments; your first one being to join the rest of us in the dining room for lunch today. We are going to leave this with you now, but if you have any questions about your itinerary we can discuss them later today."

As they left the room, Ameliah walked in.

"So, let's see it," she chirped.

"See what?"

"Uh, your schedule of course," she said bouncing onto my bed holding out her hand.

I passed her the folder Catherine had left, and pulled my knees up under my chin giving her more room. Quickly she flipped it open, turned pages, and started reading aloud.

7:00 am - Daily check in & weigh in

8:00 am - Breakfast

9:00 am - Recreation & exercise

10:00 am - Morning snack

10:40 am - Cognitive group therapy

12:00 pm - Lunch

1:00 pm - Individual therapy/chores

2:30 pm - Afternoon snack

3:15 pm - Dietary

5:00 pm - Dinner

6:00 pm - Free time/chores

7:30 pm - Evening snack

8:10 pm - Group Chat

8:45 pm - Relaxation

9:30 pm - Free time/chores

11:00 pm - Night check

"Well, at least you got a full forty-eight hours in before the bars came down," Ameliah said.

"Bars?"

"You know, like a jail. You're lucky, most newbies only get one day beforehand and you got two. Probably because you came in on Saturday, and the fact that you're a first timer for any place. Oh well, the party never lasts forever right? Welcome to reality."

She stood up putting the papers on my table, grabbed a blue cashmere sweater the colour of a robin's egg from her closet, quickly checked her hair in a mirror, and opened the door.

"I'll be back in less than an hour if you want to go to lunch together," she said, and then she disappeared.

20

In the dining room, everyone had assigned chairs on either side of a large, rectangle, oak table in correlation to their room number. Brian and Catherine sat at each end. When everyone was accounted for, Catherine called out our names to line up at a window similar to one you would find at a drive through restaurant. She then gave us cards that corresponded to our seating which we passed through the window, and in return, received a tray of food specially prepared for our own individual meal plans.

Back in my assigned chair, I kept my head down. My hair fell loosely, covering enough of my face to give me a sense of invisibility, yet enough freedom to still watch everyone else. Quickly I went around the table and calculated the differences in fat grams and caloric content of each individual plate, while silently too, observing each persons reaction to the foods presented to them. With little hesitation, every person at the table but myself, had already picked up their utensils, and started eating. I stared down at the food in front of me. A salmon sandwich on whole wheat bread, a small bowl of freshly sliced mixed fruit with cottage cheese, four ounces of vegetable juice, and eight ounces of white milk.

"Ameliah," I whispered, nudging her under the table. "Where's the nearest bathroom? I think I'm gonna be sick."

"Relax and breathe girl. No-one leaves the dining room before 12:30. House rules."

"But I really think I'm going to be sick!"

"It's just your nerves. Breathe."

"Well they really don't expect me to eat all this, do they?"

"Nah, not all of it being your first official meal and all," she whispered glancing over my tray. "But probably at least half of it."

"But there's got to be at least 750 calories here!"

At that moment, everyone at the table stopped and stared in my direction. My voice had risen and carried like the shrill of a train whistle cutting through the silence of a deserted mountain range. Before returning my eyes back to my own plate, I intentionally met every persons individual stare with a deliberate look of insolence. I thought everyone was looking at me in judgement and condemnation of my weakened outburst, when in fact, they were really empathizing with my pain and torment. Unknowingly to me at that time, every person at the table was wearing their own individual mask. The only thing separating me from them, was that they had each learned to wear their masks more freely, and more comfortably than I had.

At 12:30 a bell rang, and everyone but myself, Amy, and Catherine lined up and exited the dining room like a group of anxious third graders at the end of a school day. Ten minutes later, Amy left, and Catherine moved to the empty chair at my right.

"Jenniffer, did you read over the material we left with you earlier?"

I nodded slowly.

"Then you understand how this is going to work, yes?"

Again I nodded.

"Okay then. You have your first appointment with Dr. Burman at one o'clock, so that leaves you with one of two choices. We can sit here for the next twenty minutes and you can eat your lunch, or you can take your tray to the window and return to your room until then."

"So I'm free to go?"

"Yes Jenniffer you are free to go. But understand that if you refuse to eat your snacks and your assigned supper later today, having made no efforts on your part to co-operate by this time tomorrow, we will have no other choice but to take a more forceful course of action with your treatment at that point. Ultimately, the choice is yours how you intake your meals to meet your body's nutritional needs. The choice whether you starve yourself to death or not, is ours. You either eat, or be fed. So what's it going to be?"

I stood up, leaving my untouched tray on the table, and headed to the door.

"What happens after this next twenty four hours is up to you Jenniffer. That's something maybe you should discuss with Dr. Burman during your session." Catherine took my tray to the window, and met me in the doorway. "I'll see you here again at two thirty for snack," she said smiling. "Until then, I leave you to your decision making."

Then she walked past me and turned down the hall.

When I got back up to my room, Ameliah was there. She was speaking with someone on the phone, and from the way she jolted when I opened the door, I got the impression I was definitely interrupting something hostile. I mouthed a silent sorry, grabbed my I-pod, and sat back on my bed. Before the first track played through, Ameliah slammed down the receiver, and then the bathroom door behind her. When she came back out, I didn't want to invade her space or seem a nosy neighbour, but I couldn't help look over. She was twisting her hair into a spool, then clipped it back atop her head. When she turned to look up at the clock, I noticed her eyes were a glossed over bloodshot red.

"Don't you have your first session with Dr. Burman now?" She blared at me.

I slid off my headphones.

"Supposed to."

"Um, well then you better get moving don't you think. They're going to start getting tough on you if you don't lighten up a bit you know."

"So Catherine says."

"Well take it from someone who knows all too well girl, you've pushed it about as far as you can already." She checked her hair in the mirror over her shoulder. "Come on, I'll walk downstairs with you. I'm going out anyway."

"Can't be any worse than the last hour was," I said getting up.

"Ditto on that." she muttered.

"Hey Ameliah, are you okay?" I asked. "I don't mean to pry, it's just that...."

"Me? Okay?" She asked, putting on a clearly fake smile. "I'm fine of course. Now let's go before you're late."

The only precursor I had to any psychiatrist was that which had been portrayed to me through movies, television and books, so I couldn't help but wonder what there was anyone expected me to talk about for an hour every day.

"Hello again," Dr. Burman said, welcoming me into the office, motioning to a seating area in the centre of the room. "Please, have a seat wherever you'd like."

There was an oval, hand carved, wooden coffee table surrounded by a white, wicker rocking chair, two oversized black leather chairs, and the infamous leather sofa. I sat at the end of the sofa, closest to the door, wondering if it would make me look smaller. Dr. Burman sat in the oversized chair across from me, his pen and clipboard in hand.

"So, how are you feeling this afternoon?" He asked; his stare piercing me like an invisible sword.

I shrugged my shoulders sheepishly in answer, and Dr. Burman wrote something down.

"The first thing we need to determine," he said, "is how you would like everyone to address you. According to my notes it says that you usually go by the name Jenni by your family, friends, and peers, but you have told Catherine that your name is Jenniffer. What name would you like to be called by while you are staying here at the house?"

Silence. He wrote something down.

"I've also read in your file that you are here against your own free will, and I'm gathering from what I've seen of you so far this morning and over the last few minutes, you are not very happy about being here. Am I correct in that assumption?"

My lower back was spasming from trying to sit still, so I shifted in my seat, and then again, I shrugged him off with silence. He again scribbled something down.

"So you don't know if you are happy about being here or not?"

"I don't want to be here," I declared in a low hoarse voice. My mouth was dry, and my throat sore. "Can I please have some water?" I asked, motioning to a jug of ice water in the centre of the coffee table.

"Help yourself."

Neither of us spoke while I filled a glass with water, then put it back down without drinking. *What was I doing? This jug was probably a plant, filled with sugar water, and just placed here to trick me into ingesting even more calories.* When I pushed the glass away and sat back, Dr. Burman wrote something down.

"Okay, we've now established that you don't want to be here, which is a good start, but do you understand why you are here? Why your parents have signed you into our care?"

"Because they don't want me around causing anymore problems for them maybe," I said abruptly.

Dr. Burman looked up at me with a sudden newfound interest.

"Is that what you really think?" He asked.

"I, I guess so." I stammered. "I mean, well, maybe for them it was just easier to get rid of me for awhile rather than deal with me. Especially with everything they have to do for Steffanni's upcoming wedding. That's my little sister. She's getting married in a few weeks."

"I see. And you really believe it was easy for your parents to make the choice to institutionalize you, and then also to follow through with their decision seeing it to the end?"

"Um, well I'm here aren't I?"

"Yes, you are, and you are also...."

But 'you are also', was all I heard before I started counting. There were two small ice cubes floating in my glass of water and I looked from one to the other counting in rhythm. If one melted, I picked up the jug and poured in another.

It wasn't until Dr. Burman passed me a handful of hard covered books, that I refocused on my surroundings.

"Choose whichever one you like," he said. "If you've never done any journaling before, it may feel strange for you at first. I guarantee you though, you will soon find it a very therapeutic method of releasing your bottled up feelings and emotions."

Not really sure what he was talking about, but to appease him I chose a book with a red and black plaid cover that reminded me of a Scottish kilt, and placed the remaining ones on the sofa beside me.

"Remember, there aren't any rules when you journal. Write anytime you want, and at any length. Grammar and case don't matter. If you only want to write one word, or one thousand words, it's your choice. Feel free to draw if you like as well, and to use colour also. Anything goes. The important thing is to get the feelings out. You can choose another book when that one you have is full too, so don't hold back."

There must have been over one hundred blank pages in the book I chose, and I flipped through them quickly trying to imagine what it was he thought I had in me that I could possibly fill them with. Just then, the house bell rang, signalling it was again almost time to convene in the dining room.

"We've run a little late today," Dr. Burman said, glancing at his watch. "We can pick up from here again on Wednesday. Feel free to start writing in that journal today though."

I nodded and walked to the door.

"Dr. Burman," I said, before exiting his office. "My name is Jenniffer. I don't want it to be shortened regardless what my parents may have said. I want to be called by my full name."

"Okay then. I look forward to seeing you back here in a couple days at one o'clock Jenniffer."

He smiled, and when I turned to close the door behind me, he was writing again.

Jenniffer, I said aloud to myself while heading down the hall to the dining room. *I'm Jenniffer, not Jenni. J-E-N-N-I-F-F-E-R K-L-A-R-K . Fourteen letters.*

21

My mid afternoon snack consisted of a small dish of mixed fruit, four equally cut cheddar cheese sticks, four whole wheat crackers, and an eight ounce glass of white milk. Ameliah smiled at me when I sat down, mouthed the words good luck, and gave me the thumbs up under the table with both hands. The girl who then sat at my left, must have been outside, because when she sat down, her clothes had a noticeable air of fresh cut grass.

"Hi!," she said, setting down her tray, then extending her hand. "I'm Susan. It's really short for Susanna, but you can call me Susie if you want. You're Jenniffer right?"

I nodded, returned her smile, and shook her hand. She had a firm handshake for little fingers.

"So how long have you been sick? I hope you don't mind me asking, that is?" she questioned. "I know it's none of my business, so you don't have to tell me anything if you don't want to. It's just that you're a lot skinnier than most of us here. Even more so than some of the girls I met at other places. Well, except for this one girl I knew who weighed only sixty three pounds; I wonder what ever happened to her? Anyway, sorry, I ramble a lot. Especially in group therapy, I'm always the one doing all the talking, not that anyone else wants to, but even if they did, I never shut up. So what were we talking about? Oh yeah, so how long have you been sick?"

As Susan rambled on and on, I watched fascinated by her actions. She was like a spider spinning a web, making precise, robotic, habitual movements, roboticly without concentration. While she spoke, she took each piece of fruit from her bowl, and grouped them according to colour on a separate plate. Oranges and cantaloupes with peaches, green grapes with honeydew melon, bananas with pineapples and pears, and strawberries with cherries. Then she separated the individual fruit pieces, still in their groups, but so that not one piece was directly in contact with another. She used her knife and fork, cut her four cheese sticks into quarters, cut each quarter in half, then lined each piece around the rim of the plate, encircling her fruit sections.

"Aren't you eating?" She asked me casually, noticing I hadn't even touched my tray since setting it on the table.

"I'm not hungry."

"Look around you," she gestured around the table. "No-one else here is either, but you know what happens if you don't eat? They'll pump you full of pure liquid fat they will. As scary as tackling these trays they give us is, it's better this way. Although I guess I'm not really as scared of the food as I used to be. It's more like now I'm just scared of not knowing how much food is enough or too much because I still don't really ever feel hungry. That's where I'm learning to trust Dr. Shaw and Catherine now though. They only make enough foods available to me to sustain a healthy weight, but not enough to tempt me to overindulge. I guess I'm kind of lucky that way, that I can stop I mean. Penny, my roommate, she's out on a pass right now, and she can't help herself a lot of the time. She's a bulimic. I feel bad for her too because most days she really does try so hard not to be sick, but once she starts to eat anything she totally loses it and can't stop. She eats so fast and then goes into these panic attacks because she can't remember what she ate. Then well, you know, she throws it all up, whether she wants to or not. She actually passed out in our room one night last week after supper, all because of anxiety over what she ate; which really wasn't even that much. Imagine that. I'd never seen anyone really faint before that night, and I was really upset over it too. More so than Penny was even. Have you ever seen anybody faint before? I mean just collapse to the ground, like a deflating helium balloon hit by a bullet at top speed?"

Between her sentences, I watched Susan as she selected one item from her plate, slid it to the centre, cut it into quarters, quartered each new piece a second time, and then ate two of those pieces. When she'd eaten two pieces from each section, she placed her knife and fork in a cross formation over her plate. When the bell rang indicating that snack time was over, Susan rose simultaneously with the others.

"Well it was good talking with you Jenniffer. Maybe we can meet up in the lounge sometime and play a game of chess or something. Do you play chess?"

"My sister and I played when we were younger," I said picking up my untouched tray.

"I was on the chess team at my school before I had to go into hospital, so I'm fairly good. We could play something else though if you want to, it doesn't have to be chess. Catherine says if there is a game someone wanted to play that wasn't available, as long as they had all their privileges she'd get it for them."

I dropped my tray off at the window behind Susan and followed her out.

"I don't think I'll ever have privileges," I said.

"Sure you will," she smiled. "It's tough on everyone at first, but you will. Later," she said, waving on her way down the hall. "See you at dinner."

22

The following day after lunch, having still not touched any of the food served to me up to that point, Catherine escorted me to the medical room where I watched a short video about nasogastric feeding. When it was over, Dr. Brian Shaw joined us in the room.

"Have we come to a decision?" He asked.

I didn't answer verbally but instead climbed onto the examining table, and laid back clearing my throat. As invasive as the procedure looked, it wasn't as frightening as the thought of swallowing a tray of food. It still gave me the power to govern what I physically put in my mouth. Even if I couldn't completely control the calories they were going to force feed me, they still couldn't force me to eat.

By one thirty, I was escorted back to my room by Brian, Catherine with my new buddy pole.

"You're more stubborn than I gave you credit for," Ameliah said when we were alone. "Does it hurt?"

"My throat stings a little, and I have a headache from hell."

"Yeah, I remember I had a wicked sore throat for a couple days after my first tubing. I was pretty nauseous too. Did they give you anything for pain, or did they refuse?"

"Brian said I could have something at bedtime if I thought I really needed it."

"That's what I figured. It's one of their typical methods around here. They won't allow you anything until they feel you've suffered the cause."

"And they don't think being hooked up to this contraption is suffering enough?"

"Nope, not until you break and give in it isn't"

"Well they can shove intravenous tubes up my arm, tubes up my nose, and wherever the hell else they want for that matter, but I'm not going to break!"

Ameliah rolled her eyes and laughed.

"Oh you will break all right. Believe me, even as stubborn as you are, they will eventually get to you, and you too will give in to their demands."

"Believe me," I maintained. "I won't."

"Girl you look and sound just like I did a few months back, and trust me, you will give in."

"Well not if I have anything to say about it."

"Precisely the point Jenniffer. You don't have anything to say about it. That's why you're here dragging around that pole. You don't have those rights anymore, remember? And until you give in, that's exactly how things will remain."

I flopped down onto my bed and stared out the window. As much as I didn't want to admit it, I knew Ameliah was right. I was like a caged animal, imprisoned to be completely retrained before I would be set free.

Due to my relentless unwillingness to cooperate voluntarily in the program, over the next few days I lost all of what were considered my house privileges. I was prohibited from having any visitors or use of the telephone. I wasn't allowed computer time or free time in the lounge or anywhere outside on the grounds. I wasn't allowed to participate in any form of physical exercise that could be construed as a form of weight loss, however I was permitted to participate in the relaxation and yoga group. As far as socializing with any of the other guests, I wasn't permitted in their rooms, but because Ameliah had privileges they were allowed in our room during free time, but not supposed to socialize with me. If they were caught, they received a warning the first time, and the second time would lose their privileges then too, so we were always careful to whisper. To gain any of my privileges meant only one thing; giving in to the demands and restrictions put upon me. In the lounge each guest had an assigned mailbox with a large cubby hole underneath, and mine was the only one with something unclaimed in it. In order to receive the contents in my mailbox, I would have to attend weigh ins and stand on the scale each morning without any fuss or objections.

On my twelfth day of nasogastic and intravenous fluids, I knew I had gained weight. What I couldn't tell from looking in the mirror was exactly how much weight I'd gained, and it was beginning to scare me. So the next morning, I decided I would find out how much fat this thing was actually putting into me, let them weigh me, and in return be allowed to collect my mail. At seven a.m. sharp, I lined up with the rest of the guests outside the medical room, and waited anxiously in turn to be called.

When I entered the room, I was met by Catherine, Amy, and Dr. Shaw. Amy led me behind a curtain, and handed me an olive green, cotton, polyester gown similar to something you would see a patient wearing while walking around in a hospital. The only difference being that this gown had velcro closures up the sides, instead of ties.

"Change into this, removing all your other clothing as quickly as you can, Jenniffer. Then meet us at the scale when you're ready," Amy said.

After a bit of a struggle getting around my intravenous tubing, I walked over to where the three of them were standing. Dr. Shaw first took my blood pressure, my temperature, and then asked me to stretch my arms as high as I could into the air, and hold the position. I didn't know why he wanted me to this, but I followed his instructions. Amy then waved a small black wand up from the outside of my left foot, over top of me, down to my right foot, and then completely around me. I felt like a criminal ready to be strip searched for smuggling something across an international border.

"What are you doing?" I asked sharply.

"Checking for weights," Catherine replied. "You can put your arms back down at your sides and relax now, Jenniffer."

Then Dr. Shaw felt my stomach, and listened to it with his stethoscope.

"Don't tell me," I said sarcastically. "Now you're checking for a baby under all my fat right?"

"No, Jenniffer," Catherine said again certainly unamused. "We're making sure you haven't water loaded weight before coming in."

When Dr. Shaw instructed me next to get onto the scale, I drew in a deep breath, and stepped up.

"Turn around please Jenniffer, so that your back is to the bar," Dr. Shaw said firmly.

I turned, unimpressed, and listened to the small weighted bars being slid back and forth across the scale, then after a minute all slid back to one side.

"You can step down, and get redressed now," Dr. Shaw said.

When I hesitated, Catherine gestured back toward the curtain, and thanked me for my cooperation. I changed as speedily as I could, and went back out to join them.

"Where should I put this?" I asked, holding up the gown.

"You can drop it in the bin beside the door with the rest of them on your way out," Amy said. "I'll show you."

"That's it then?" I asked.

"For now," Catherine said smiling. "I'll make sure you get your mail after breakfast."

"Okay, well thanks," I said slowly. I followed Amy to the door, and then turned back to Catherine and Dr. Shaw questioningly. "But aren't you going to tell me how much I weigh?"

"No," Catherine answered. "I'm sorry, but we can't."

"What do you mean, you can't?"

"I'm sorry, Jenniffer. That is our policy."

"But that's not fair!" I shouted. "It's my body! What gives you the right to know how much I weigh, and not me?"

Catherine's answer was straightforward, and left no room for me to argue.

"Your parents' signature," was all she said.

23

After stomping up the stairs back to my room, I climbed directly back under the still warm blankets on my bed.

"Hey, what's with all the attitude?" Ameliah asked. "I heard you thumping that pole of yours all the way up the stairs."

"Why didn't you tell me before I went down there that they weren't going to tell me how much weight I've gained?"

"Oh, that," she said. "Sorry, I never really thought about it."

"What do you mean you never thought about it? How the hell can you not think about it? It's all I ever think about!"

"Sorry, you just get used to it after awhile I guess."

"I can't imagine ever getting that used to any of this," I sighed, sinking further into my pillow.

"Well I have. You kind of stop caring altogether after awhile. About everything."

It wasn't only what Ameliah said that made me turn to her, it was her tone. As I remained comfortably in my bed, I watched Ameliah walk around the perimeter of her bed. She meticulously smoothed each sheet on her bed flat, tugging and folding the edges into perfect hospital corners. After her initial beauty, that was the one thing about Ameliah that everyone noticed which was that she was always making sure everything was always just so, and in its specified, proper place. Everything always had to be perfect.

This particular morning however, it was Ameliah's mannerisms that seemed standoffish. When she caught me watching her, she shot me her brightest, widest, steward smile. However, it was her eyes that caught my attention. Her smile was flashy but her eyes had lost their sparkle. I didn't see sadness or anger; just indifference. Her eyes seemed empty of any true emotion like she really had stopped caring.

Before I got the words out to ask her what was so wrong, there was a loud knock at the door, and without waiting as always, Susie quickly rushed in, followed by Penny.

"Hey you," Susie, greeted me, bouncing onto my bed. "What are you doing tucked in again? Aren't you going to the dining room? You know, if it makes you feel any better, they won't let any of us know what are weights are."

"Yeah, they say it can have too much of a negative influence on our recovery if we knew," said Penny. "Especially with those of us that have a major compulsion with competition."

"That's you all right Penny," jested Susie. "Wasn't it last week you were on a kick about looking like Tweety Bird? Comparing yourself to the looks of fictional cartoon characters. Even for you that was a new one."

Penny was finishing crisscrossing the ends of Ameliah's hair into a long French braid when the breakfast bell rang a minute later. With her hair pulled back away from her face, the emptiness in Ameliah's eyes, was now even more apparent to me than before.

"Do you want me to tell Catherine that you have a migraine and not feeling well or something?" Ameliah asked. "Tell her that's the reason you're not in the dining room."

"You can tell her anything you want," I said angrily. "I really don't care."

"Sure you don't. I'll tell her you have a bad headache, and it's making you feel nauseous. Then maybe at least she will still let you get your mail."

"Yeah, we'll vouch for you too," Susie said nudging Penny's arm. "Right?"

"Sure," said Penny. "See you later."

I didn't take my eyes off the clock after Ameliah shut the door behind the three of them, and at ten after eight, Catherine walked in.

"You're not in the dining room," she said. "How come?"

"Because I'm here, in bed," I struck back, flipping over onto my other side to face the wall away from her.

She walked around to face me again.

"Some of the other girls said you have migraine headache, but I can't help to wonder if that is the actual truth, or if they're just covering for you because you would rather lay here and sulk over weigh-ins, rather than adhere to the rules, and join the rest of us for breakfast."

I glared up at her.

"What? So my friends here are all liars now, is that it?"

She didn't retaliate, but just stood in front of me suddenly grinning like a player about to checkmate his unsuspecting opponent. This only infuriated me more, but confused me somewhat also.

"What is so amusing?" I asked sharply.

"That you have friends here," she said smugly, dropping my mail on my desk beside me before then heading back toward the door. "And to think, you thought you were all alone."

When the door clicked shut behind her, I stuck my middle finger up at it, then swung my feet over the side of my bed, and grabbed the three envelopes she had left. I quickly tore into the first one without looking at the postmark.

My Dearest Jenni,

Your father and I want you to know that our love and prayers are with you every minute, of every day. We know that you were very angry with us the last time we saw you, but we hope you understand that we did what we thought was best for you. Steffanni also sends her love, and says to reassure you that she will not get married without her big sister at her side to share in her day. Your father and I have been discussing your progress with the Shaws' regularly, and are happy to hear that you are finally gaining some of your strength back. Both Catherine and Brian have assured us that they are making certain all your needs are being met, and that we should be able to come and visit you very soon. Until then, please take care of yourself Jenni, and know how much we all love and miss you. I've enclosed some postage stamps so you can write, but please call us as soon as you have your telephone privileges so that we can talk regularly. We all look very forward to hearing from you soon, and the day you can come home back to us.

Lots of love,
Mom & Dad

"Garbage!" I said, letting the papers, stamps and all, drop into the waste basket. Before opening the second envelope, I turned it over and checked for a return address. It was from the Café.

Our Sweet Jenniffer,

We all miss you here at the café tremendously, and you have many loyal customers who inquire daily as to your prospective return, who also wish you well. Cindy is the only one here who knows your true whereabouts as I haven't said anything to anyone else. I didn't think it was anyone else's business knowing the personal details of your ailments, or that you would want anyone knowing either. I've simply said that you are away on sick leave, and left it at that.

Ken wants me to tell you not to worry at all about things here with us. He says to reassure you that your position is completely secure, and that it will be here waiting for you when you are well enough to resume your duties, regardless of the time frame. That means not to rush your treatment Jenniffer. Your health and well being are the most important things right now, and need to remain your top priority, as they are our only concern.

I called Caitlynne's Place last week to speak with you, but the lady who answered said you couldn't receive calls yet. She sounded friendly enough, gave me your address so we could write, and said I could call and check in on your progress also at any time with your mom's permission. I hope you will write back and let us hear from you personally about how you are really doing. Also, if there is anything that Ken or myself can do for you, or anything that you might need or want that we can send you to make your stay there more comfortable, please let us know. Cindy also said you could call her at anytime you felt like talking, and that she too will visit when she can.

Your road ahead will no doubt be a difficult one for you Jenniffer, but remember you are not alone on your journey. We are all here for you. Keep strong Jenniffer, and do whatever you have to do to get yourself better and back home to us.

Love and Best Wishes,
Mrs. Mary-Anne Walker

The third envelope was a shimmering white, larger than the first two, and beautifully embossed with two entwined lilies climbing up the left side. Paper clipped to the inside of a matching invitation to Steffanni's wedding, was a brief note scrawled in Steffanni's handwriting.

Sis,
There's no return attendance card, because I already know you will be there standing beside me.
Much Love & Laughter,
Steffi.

I carefully tucked the wedding invitation and the letter from Mary-Anne into the top drawer of my desk, and got up. I stood tall, and studied my reflection in the mirror twisting and turning looking from side to side. The more I looked, the more clearly I could see it. It was in my face, in my legs, my behind, most definitely my stomach, and even in my hands. It was sheer fat; through and through. I had definitely gained weight, and I had to know how much. I counted the days on my fingers until Staffani's wedding, and panicked at the thought. It was now only eight weeks away.

Looking at the clock, sure I hadn't missed the bell signalling the end of breakfast, I snuck out of my room and back down the stairs to the medical room. The door was locked tight. Not ready to give up on my quest, and positive there had to be another scale somewhere in the house, I searched room to room trying to find one with no luck. I did however, find Brian and Catherine's door unlocked, and once inside found something even more valuable than a scale. On top of a sitting table I found the clipboard with everyone's weigh-in sheets from earlier that morning.

Quickly losing track of time, I flipped through the sheets scanning each one briefly in search of my name. They weren't in alphabetical order, but listed instead by room number. Suddenly feeling a little nauseous, I sat down on a wooden chest at the foot of the Shaws' bed, and started to read.

By the time I was aware of the voices gathering in the hallway or had a chance to hide, Catherine was standing before me..

"Jenniffer!" She exclaimed. "How did you get in here? More importantly though, what the heck are you doing in here in the first place?"

She walked across the room stopping directly in front of me. I stood up alarmed by her soldier like stance, and tried to slip the clipboard under the back of my shirt.

"I, I ...."

"You what? And what is that you have behind your back?" She reached around me and snatched the clipboard out of my hands. "How much of this did you read?"

I didn't speak.

"Well," she demanded, waving the charts in front of my face like a geisha girl fanning her prince. "How much?"

"Only enough to know that you lied to me about how fat all these things are making me!" I screamed back at her, pointing to the tube taped to the side of my nose. I looked past her at the group of girls being shown away from the door by Dr. Shaw, then grabbed my pole and bolted through them all, up the stairs, and into my bathroom.

After a few minutes of silence, Ameliah knocked softly on the door.

"Jenniffer?"

I looked straight ahead of me into the mirror, completely repulsed by my own reflection, while tear stained cheeks and darkened eyes looked back at me from the mirror. Unable to answer Ameliah, or move away, I stood still, as if frozen by my own fear of what I'd become. I was trapped in my own reflection.

Just eighteen more pounds, I mouthed. *The nine they've made you gain back, then nine more to ensure safety from them. Then you will be okay again.* I wiped my face dry with the back of my sleeve. *Lose those eighteen more pounds and then you can stop. Just eighteen more pounds okay,* I whispered to the girl in the mirror. *Another eighteen pounds and then you will finally be happy.*

Ameliah knocked on the door again.

"Hey Jenniffer, are you okay in there?"

"No," I called out flatly. "But don't worry. I will be."

Then without further hesitation, I drew in one long, deep breath, counted to fourteen, and pulled my nasogastric and intravenous tubes both completely out.

24

My nose was still bleeding a little when I finally left the bathroom. Penny and Susan were standing with Ameliah at her desk, and they all stopped talking, and turned when I opened the door. Trying to avoid them, I put my head down, and hurried past leaving my unattached pole and tubes in the bathroom. All three of them followed me to my side of the room like a gaggle of geese on water. When I hopped up onto my bed, they surrounded me, and Ameliah grabbed my chin, twisting my face up to hers.

"My God woman! You pulled out your tubes?"

I slapped her hand away.

"So what if I did?"

"Shit lady, maybe you are just crazy after all."

"There was this girl at Linwood County, the first hospital I was in," Susan said speedily, gaining our attention. "She had a really violent side to her too, though. I remember this one time, she threw an entire tray of food at this nurse just because the nurse opened a package of salad dressing and poured it onto the girl's lettuce. Of course the girl was right to get mad about her food being touched and all, but, well anyway, that girl, she pulled her tubes out so many times, she learned how to put them back in again all by herself. The nurses would hook her up, and then wonder why she wasn't gaining any weight. Boy, when they finally caught on to what she was doing, did she ever get it. They went and hooked her right up to hyper after that they did. Come to think of it now, I don't really remember seeing her after that because they moved her upstairs to intensive or something shortly thereafter."

"What is hyper?" I asked, accepting a Kleenex from a hesitant Ameliah.

For a minute, all three of them were quiet. Even Susan seemed somehow lost for words, which I didn't think was possible. They looked back and forth to each other exchanging what looked like fearful glances like three sisters caught in the act of coming home late past curfew, and neither one the courage to speak.

"Hyper is short for hyperalimentation," Penny finally spoke out, breaking the silence. "It's when they cut a hole in your chest and surgically put the tubes inside you. Then you can't just pull them out."

Penny pulled down the collar of her shirt, revealing a small, nickel sized scar.

"They had you on hyper before you came here?" Susan questioned Penny with heartfelt concern.

"The last three weeks I was there."

"You never told me. Was it as painful as they say it is?"

"Well the first week I think I was pretty out of it, but then after that it wasn't too bad I guess. The rapid weight gain and all was the worst part, not the incision."

"Speaking of which," Ameliah cut in abruptly. "How much weight have you gained lately Jenniffer? Or better yet, why don't you tell us all how much we've all gained?"

It was obvious that Ameliah was referring to me finding and reading the charts, but I tried to play unaware and casual nonetheless.

"How the hell should I know?" I retorted.

"Oh please. Penny saw you with the charts in your hand just a few minutes ago. Downstairs after you broke into the Shaws' quarters she saw and heard you with Catherine in her bedroom. You had the charts in your hand."

"Okay girls, break it up now," Catherine ordered walking in. "If you three girls wouldn't mind leaving the room for a few minutes," she said signalling to Penny, Susan, and Ameliah. "I would like to speak to Jenniffer alone."

"Sure," said Ameliah. "But not until she answers my question."

"No," Catherine said firmly. "Now please."

"Why should I have to leave when this is my room too?" Asked Ameliah angrily.

Catherine didn't have to say anything else. The look in her eyes said it all as she stared the three girls down like a rabid wolf stalking a helpless litter of rabbits in a patch of clover.

"Oh fine," Ameliah huffed following Penny and Susan to the door. "But this isn't over yet roomy."

When Catherine turned her attention back to me, I don't think she realized at first the extent of my mornings events. I watched her gaze as she searched my face, my arms, and then my face with her eyes a second time. When she noticed my tubes were gone, her face turned as red as a hothouse tomato, and I was sure she was going to pop a blood vessel, if she hadn't already. After looking around the room, and then the bathroom, she collected my discards and made her way back to the door.

"Put on something warm for outside, and meet me in the front lobby in ten minutes," she said. Then she turned, and walked out closing the door tightly behind her.

Had I made her so furious with me that she was going to kick me out of the program? Could she even do that I wondered, without having my parents' permission? It was her program after all, and it was her home. Eagerly I jumped up and grabbed my navy cardigan off the back of my desk chair, and pulled it around my shoulders.

Finally, I thought, I was taking my first step back to freedom. I was finally getting out of here.

25

At the bottom of the stairway, Catherine was speaking with Brian and Dr. Burman who each gave me a friendly smile as I walked up to them. Catherine had a large manilla envelope and a burgundy leather bound book tucked under her arm that reminded me of a large Bible my grandmother used to own.

"Ready?" She asked me.

I nodded, trying not to look too overjoyed at the thought of going home.

"Let's not waste any more time then," she said turning toward the lobby.

I stepped out onto the porch ahead of her. It was the first time I'd been outdoors since my arrival, and I deeply breathed in the fresh air like a drowning child pulled from the sea. The sun was shining brightly in a cloudless summer sky, casting the perfect amount of heat to compliment the steady breeze, rustling the leaves on the surrounding trees.

I followed Catherine around to the back of the house in silence, then along the path winding through the trees behind that lead to the pond and waterfall. It was refreshing to be walking outdoors, and when I escaped this place and finally got home, I told myself, the first thing I was going to do was go for a long walk along the river behind the Café.

"Why don't we stop here and rest for awhile," Catherine said, sitting on a bench arriving at the clearing under the large willow. "It will give us a chance to talk."

As I sat down beside her, it was obvious to me that the bench had been hand carved with caring craftsmanship, and I couldn't resist sliding my fingers loosely through the rounded spirals that framed the side.

"My husband made this bench for me almost ten years ago," Catherine said.

"Brian? Dr. Shaw made this himself?"

Catherine nodded.

"I've never seen a bench so detailed before. He must have spent hours carving all of this."

"He did. It was a very therapeutic project for him after our daughter passed away."

"You two had a daughter?" I asked surprised.

"Yes," she smiled. "And this place here, where we are sitting now, was her most favourite spot on these entire grounds. She used to come out here and sit for hours upon hours, just sketching and writing poetry. She was a very bright and talented young lady our Caitlynne."

"Your daughter's name was Caitlynne?"

"It was. She passed ten years ago."

"I am so sorry. How did she die? I mean, if it's not too personal?"

"It's not. Actually, that is why I wanted to bring you out here to talk. You remind me and Brian a lot of our daughter you know. Especially of the last few weeks she was with us before we lost her to her anorexia."

"You mean your daughter died from dieting?"

"If you wish to refer to it like that, then yes, she did."

"Oh my gosh. How old was she?"

"Officially seventeen." Catherine brushed the tips of her fingers lightly across a small copper plate mounted into the back of the bench. "CAITLYNNE MARIE SHAW - 1977 - 1994" She had her whole life ahead of her, our Caitlynne did. She was intelligent, talented, very beautiful, and incredibly strong willed. Just like you are Jenniffer."

"But I still don't understand? How did she actually die?"

"Well eventually, after months of purging, and the up and down fluctuating of scales, her organs couldn't keep up with the demands and restraints she was putting on her body. She didn't have the nutrients to keep her organs functioning properly. First, her liver swelled to the size of a football, her kidneys shut down, and then her heart gave in, all in a matter of hours. She went into full cardiac arrest trying to do sit ups in bed three days before her eighteenth birthday."

Catherine continued talking, letting her tears roll freely from her eyes to her chin, dropping silently to her lap.

"Brian and I laid our daughter to rest, finally at peace, on the day of her eighteenth birthday."

"That must have been so difficult for you," I gasped. "I can't even imagine anything so horrible!"

"Ah but Jenniffer, isn't that why you are here now?" She motioned around the property. "Here, with all of us at Caitlynne's Place?"

I rubbed my arms, suddenly feeling chilled.

"You are twenty-eight now, correct?" Catherine asked.

I didn't move.

"What you need to ask yourself Jenniffer, is whether you want to live to see your twenty-ninth birthday, or die at twenty-eight?"

I looked up at her, startled by her statement. Then she passed me the burgundy leather bound book she had been carrying with her. It was a scrapbook, filled with pages of photographs depicting the final years of a young girls life.

"And if you choose to live," Catherine said raising the cover, "Is this the quality of life you want to sustain?"

The first photograph was of a young girl standing beside Dr. Shaw, wearing a full length fuchsia prom dress.

"That is Caitlynne," Catherine said, pointing to the picture. "It was taken at her sweet sixteen party."

"She looks like you."

Catherine smiled proudly, then flipped to the last photo.

"And that picture was taken the day before she died."

"No way? That's her?" I asked, lifting the book for a closer look.

The girl in the second picture didn't look anything like the girl in the first photograph, except that she was wearing the same fuchsia dress. In this picture though, the dress looked many sizes too big, and hung loosely like a heavy wet drape over a thin drying rack.

"She looks like a run down cancer patient," I said soberly. "I mean, she's so thin and everything. I would never have recognized her in this picture if you hadn't told me it was her."

"My daughter weighed ninety-six pounds when that picture was taken. And how much do you weigh right now?"

I didn't answer.

"Oh come now Jenniffer. You just read it on your chart a little over an hour ago. I know you remember. You weigh ninety-six pounds, right?"

"I read it, but ...."

"But what? You don't think you look like that, do you?" Catherine flipped back to the first photograph in the book again. "You see yourself more like my Caitlynne does there, don't you? Except you probably think you still need to lose a few more pounds before you will look that good for your sisters' wedding, right?"

"I just need to lose eighteen more pounds," I said under my breath.

Catherine turned back to the last photograph again, paused, and then closed the book. Then she took my hand in hers, and pushed my palm flat over the copper plate on the back of the bench.

"Lose eighteen more pounds Jenniffer, and you will look like that."

I jerked my hand away.

"There are six other benches on the property similar to this one. Each one of them dedicated to another victim of an eating disorder that stayed here at Caitlynne's Place, who also in the end, lost their own life in battle with this relentless disease. Do you really want to be benched at age twenty-eight?"

I looked up at her, my own tears now making their way to my chin.

"I don't want to die if that's what you mean, but I don't want to live like this anymore either."

"Like what?"

"Ugly! Fat!"

"But that's just it Jenniffer. You are nowhere near fat. You weigh only ninety-six pounds!"

"Then why can I feel it?" I cried. "Why when I look in the mirror are ugly and fat all that I see? Everywhere! All over me! Hanging off me like a sagging cow sack?" I smacked my stomach and legs. "Look at this! It's disgusting! I am disgusting!"

"Mirror image, Jenniffer. Right now you are seeing things distorted. You are a mere shell of skin and bones but you see fat where there isn't any. Combined with the chemical imbalance in your body, it is what you've conditioned yourself to see."

"That makes no sense. Why would I condition myself to see fat when all I want is to be thin?"

"Give it time Jenniffer. This is something we will cover with you in our dietary classes, as well as in the cognitive group with Dr. Burman. As time goes by, I think you will be pleasantly surprised to realize that all is not really what you see. The same as you are now realizing that you are not as alone in your struggles as you once thought and felt also. Correct?"

"Okay well yes, you were right about that one. I haven't felt completely alone since meeting Ameliah and some of the others I guess."

"You and Ameliah have become quite good friends over the past couple weeks it seems."

"You have no idea. I'd be so lost without her here to talk to. She is younger than me by a few years but she understands me. Really understands me. I don't know what I'm going to do when she leaves to go home for good."

"You realize that day may be coming sooner than you think?"

"I know. I saw her chart with mine. We can be pen pals though, and we can talk over the phone, and she can come visit me here too right? She can still come here to visit after she's been discharged can't she?"

"She can if she wants to, and if you have that privilege."

I looked away. To get that privilege of having visitors meant I would have to eat fifteen hundred calories a day; voluntarily. Catherine looked at her watch, and stood up.

"I think it's time we head back and join the others again. How about it?"

"I guess that means I'm not going home today then, doesn't it?"

"In time Jenniffer. Healing of all things takes time, and until you are strong enough mentally as well as physically to be on your own and take good care of yourself, we are going to do it for you."

"I thought you were going to kick me out of your house," I said standing.

"You mean you were hoping." Catherine said, looking back at me with a hint of a chuckle. "I don't give up on people that easily Jenniffer. And by the way, after group Dr. Shaw and I will be reinserting your tubes. And Jenniffer, if you pull them out a second time, believe me, we will put you on hyperalimentation feeding."

I followed Catherine back along the path toward the house, noticing this time, another bench at the opening entry. I didn't stop and take the time to read the name on the small plaque, even though I wanted to. I wanted to find out everything I could about these other people that Catherine said had also actually died from dieting. I wanted to know how, and needed to know why?

26

Everyone was seated in a circle of chairs when Catherine and I entered the recreation room, and they all stared when the door opened.

"Welcome, Jenniffer, Catherine," Dr. Burman greeted us cordially as Catherine pulled up two chairs to join in the circle. "We were just going around the room checking in to see how everyone is doing this morning," Dr. Burman continued. "Susan, I believe you were just about to share something with the group?"

"I'm Susie, and right now I'm feeling very frustrated," Susan spoke freely.

"What has you frustrated this morning, Susan?"

"Jenniffer," she said matter of factly demanding my attention. "I'm frustrated because she knows what my weight is and I don't. It's not fair. I'm not really angry about it or anything though because I really like Jenniffer. She's a really nice lady when you get to know her, and I think we all understand why she did what she did, sneaking around and all. I still don't think it's fair though, that she read my chart and I can't." Susan let out an exasperated sigh, shrugging her shoulders.

"I see," said Dr. Burman. "And does anyone else feel the same as Susan regarding this situation?"

Everyone in the room, but the girl sitting beside me, including Ameliah, nodded in agreement. I hung my head in guilt and shame.

"Kerrie?" Dr. Burman questioned the girl sitting beside me, "What are your feelings about Jenniffer's behaviour this morning?"

"I don't know what she did," the girl said hardly moving her lips.

"Well then maybe this would be a good opportunity for Jenniffer to check in, and she can explain for herself about her actions."

I looked to Catherine for reprieve, but she wasn't expressing any visible signs of leniency. She only nodded gesturing me to begin, as did Dr. Burman who pen in hand as always, was surely waiting to scribble down all the details of my latest defiance in my own words to use against me later.

I wanted to be tough. I wanted everyone in the room to see me as someone to be reckoned with. Someone that could always hold her own and not be pushed around. Someone who neither Catherine, Brian, nor Dr. Burman could break, regardless. When I looked around the room though, in the faces of the others, I could see the same emotions and desires as in myself. Rebounding back to me, was fear, anger, helplessness, and something unexpected; compassion. I started to cry, weeping uncontrollably like a remorseful child.

"I'm sorry," I cried. "I wasn't trying to upset everybody. I didn't care what anybody else weighed, and I still don't. No, I mean, I don't not care about any of you, just that I don't care what any of you weigh or anything. I just wanted to know how much I weigh. I needed to know how much weight I've gained from my tubes."

Catherine passed me a tissue, and I somehow managed to stop my flow of tears.

"You don't have your pole? You got your tubes out even after you broke so many rules?" Elizabeth asked seemingly confused.

"The crazy bitch pulled them out," Ameliah stated. "She left them in our sink."

"Well they are going back in again later if that makes you happy," I blurted.

"Your tubes. Your business." Interjected Susan. "I just think we should all get to know our weight since you do. It's only fair."

"But Susie I don't know what you weigh! Yes I broke into the Shaws' rooms and found the charts but honestly, I don't remember hardly anything. I was angry, and scared, and desperate, and I didn't even really understand half of what I was looking at. I'm sorry okay." I glanced up at Ameliah who was sitting directly across from me. "The only person's chart I remember anything about is Ameliah's," I said hesitantly. "Everyone else's is a blur."

"Well I forgive her," Susan chirped. "Cause I know how that kind of desperation can make you act. I'm still frustrated by all of it though, even if you don't remember my stats Jenniffer." She looked to Dr. Burman. "Is that wrong for me to still feel that way, even if I've forgiven her?"

"Your feelings are your feelings Susan," Dr. Burman replied. "And in no ways can your feelings be right or wrong. It is what you do with those feelings; how you choose to act upon them that becomes the right or wrong."

"But that's not true either," Elizabeth interjected flatly.

"Why do you say that?" Dr. Burman asked with a look of curiosity.

"Because of how I feel about food."

"I'm not following your thought Elizabeth. Could you elaborate further for all of us?"

"Well, it's like all you Dr.'s keep telling me, if I continue with my own eating patterns, I will die. I know logically that if I eat I will live, but I truly feel that with every bite of food I take, I will surely die. Therefore, my feelings aren't right, they are wrong. Even without action."

"Not exactly. Let's examine that a little more closely. It's not really those feelings you're having that are right or wrong Elizabeth, it's your perception that's misconstrued. Because of the chemical imbalance an eating disordered person suffers due to their malnourished body, their perception of reality, what is true, and what is fiction is greatly impaired. So it isn't specifically the feelings your having that are wrong, it's the chemical imbalances causing the thought patterns we need to keep working on. The feeling is the result of the negative thought. It is the thought that is wrong."

"Kind of like an alcoholic off the wagon," Penny said. "But instead of in a drunken stupor, we're in a malnourished disillusionment."

"Good analogy, Penny. Yes."

"Well if I had a choice between the two," Valerie said. "I think I'd rather be an alcoholic than an anorectic any day."

"Why is that?" Asked Dr. Burman, writing frantically as usual.

"Because food is everywhere. The temptation is all the time, and there is no way to ever get around that. It doesn't matter where you are, or what you're doing; the food is always a factor. It's always in your face."

"And you don't think that alcoholics have to fight that same battle of resisting their urges and temptations to drink?"

"Sure. But at least it's not thrown in their face every hour, every minute, of every day. They at least get a choice whether to drink or not, or whether they walk past or into the liquor store and buy that next bottle of booze. An anorectic can't just make that choice, we're forced against our will."

"Exactly," said Penny. "We can't just take a different route to avoid our drug of choice like an alcoholic can the liquor store. We have to go into the grocery store. We are force fed our drug."

"True to a point," said Dr. Burman. "But recovery from any addiction is a choice, regardless the drug. Alcoholic or anorectic, you do still have choices."

"Yeah right," mumbled Kerrie beside me. "Sure we do."

Turning toward her, nodding in agreement, I noticed first her forearms, and then her hands. Her arms were covered in scars and scratch marks that reminded me of an old leather chair once used as a feline scratching post. Her fingers extended from her hands like thin spindly branches on a small barren tree, and her nails were cut back so short at the ends, that the tips of her fingers were exposed.

As the group continued with their discussion around me, I now couldn't take my eyes off Kerrie's hands, bewildered and spellbound by their movements. Her right hand was cupped over the top of her left, and she continuously dragged her right thumb back and forth, over and through the top layer of skin on the back of her left hand. Every time droplets of blood rose to the surface, she smeared them over like a child finger-painting her hands with red paint.

When I looked up at her, she reminded me of one of those people you see on talk shows they put in a hypnotic trance to do funny things. Only this wasn't funny. Kerrie's eyes were wide like an owls at night, focussed too on her hands, and while I watched her, I didn't see her blink once. It was obvious that she was hurting herself, and although they were only surface cuts, she still showed no sign of pain. She didn't even wince. I couldn't help but wonder if she was even aware in that moment of what she was doing to herself, she was so concentrated. Did she even know where she was, or had she gone to that same distant place I went to when I binged? That place where time seemed to stand still, and awareness of anything around me was void. Watching her, I wondered if this girl would remember anything that was said in the group, or even know when she snapped back into reality, why she had blood on her fingers, and the back of her hand.

When Dr. Burman called out her name, Kerrie jerked back in her chair like someone waking suddenly out of a bad dream, and looked up.

"We're checking out now Kerrie. Is there anything you would like to add or say about today's session before we end for lunch?"

"I don't think so," she said, stretching her sleeves down over her hands. "Except that, I don't really think it matters what a persons drug of choice is when it comes to addiction. Be it drugs, alcohol, food or whatever. We're all walking the same self destructing tightrope. In the end, does it really matter how we all got to the bottom, when it's where we all ended up? It's all the same right?"

When she finished, she turned to me and forced a weak smile signalling she was done, and it was my turn again to speak. I didn't comment on anything anyone else had said, but simply reaffirmed that I was sorry again for going through the morning charts.

It was eleven forty when the group let out, and Catherine pulled me aside giving me two choices. I was to either go to the dining room at twelve o'clock and take in my lunch orally with everyone else, or I was to meet her and Dr. Shaw in the medical room in the next five minutes to have my intravenous and nasogastric tubes relined. Catherine didn't wait around to listen to my questions, excuses, or hear my answer. She just matter of fact stated that she would see me in one room or the other at the said time, and walked away down the hall.

I met her in the medical room at exactly eleven forty five.

27

At one o'clock I dragged my new pole downstairs to Dr. Burman's office for my individual therapy session. The entire way down I was preparing myself for what I thought was going to be a lecture about my recent behaviours and the groups' reactions. To my surprise, the thing Dr. Burman wanted to discuss with me was whether or not I had started to journal. When I told him I still hadn't written anything yet, he again expressed his position as to what a powerful and healing coping tool journaling was, and the significance it could have in my recovery. I agreed to try and write or draw something in my book later that day, even though I still felt I had nothing worth wasting paper to say. That's when Dr. Burman caught me completely off guard. I still don't know why, but for some reason, whether it was something he said, or the way he looked at me, I confided in him about the numbers in my head. I knew I was going to regret it later terribly, but in that moment, I found myself freely explaining to him how I was always so preoccupied by the numbers, and especially whenever I became stressed or anxious about something. I also admitted that for some reason, unknown to me, I always focussed on the number fourteen. He didn't agree with me that this was crazy. He said it was symptomatic. Then again he changed the subject.

"Why don't you tell me how you felt after leaving the cognitive group session this morning."

"It was okay I guess," I shrugged.

"The question was how did you feel, Jenniffer?"

How did I feel? What kind of a question was that?

"I don't know," I said. "I don't think I really felt anything after.. I don't know if I know how to really feel anymore. Anything good that is I mean."

"I see." He said, pausing and writing for what seemed a long, drawn out period of time. "One of the advantages of attending a group like that is to help you rediscover your feelings in a safe environment in which you can relate to your peers, and they can relate to you. Although every one of you here in this house are at different places in your recoveries, you are essentially all in the same boat. Each and every one of you can relate and understand what the other is going through, whereas those outside of these walls can't relate at all to your struggles. Although this support is crucial, it is also however just as important not to alienate your outside support systems in the process."

"I don't have any outside support systems," I stated coldly.

"Your family is an outside support system."

"I don't have any family."

Dr, Burman wrote.

"There must be someone you can think of that you have for support that you talk to."

"Well I guess I do still have my sister, but I can't talk to her right now, being on restriction. And she really doesn't understand anyway. I can talk to Ameliah though."

Dr. Burman got up and walked over behind his desk, flipped over some pages in a file, and then returned to his seat, all without putting down his clipboard. He must have been afraid I would snatch it and read what he'd been writing about me if he did.

"Ameliah is your roommate?"

I nodded.

"And she is younger than you, if I recall? Almost five years; yes?"

"About that, I think."

"And the two of you have become quite good friends in the time you've shared here so far?"

"I guess. I talk to Penny and Susan sometimes too when they come into our room to visit Ameliah. I haven't really had the chance to get to know anyone else except in groups and the dining room. It's hard to get to know people when you're on complete restriction you know."

"But you do talk to some of the others?"

"Not like Ameliah."

"What kind of things do you and Ameliah talk about when you're together?"

"Well nothing bad, if that's what you're wondering," I said, knowing it was. I could see it in his face. Concern. He wanted to know if Ameliah and I were competing with each other like Susie and Penny did. I could tell he didn't want to come right out and ask me directly either. He wanted me to volunteer the information freely to him like I had told him about the numbers in my head.

"We're not comparing ourselves to each other or trading secrets, if that's what you're concerned about," I said.

"Why do you think I am concerned?"

"You mean you're not?" I was puzzled. "You don't care about that?"

"I never said I didn't care."

"But you looked, I mean, I just assumed that was what you were thinking."

"Never assume anything, Jenniffer. Especially that of another's thoughts."

"Well why else would you be questioning me about my friendship with Ameliah if you weren't worried that we were toxic for eachother in some way?"

"I ask questions because that is my job. It is how I get to know you, and what you are all about."

"Why?"

"So that I can understand you, and ultimately help you."

"Oh for Pete's sake. Why does everyone keep saying that. I don't need any help!"

"If you really believe that you don't need help Jenniffer, then why do you think you are here?"

"Why? Because my parents betrayed, and abandoned me here on the Shaws' doorstep, that's why. Dumped me like an unwanted, runt puppy in a farmer's field."

"I see," he said raising an eyebrow, writing.

"My God," I huffed. "Don't you people ever give up?"

"No."

I looked up at the clock and started counting off the seconds, fourteen at a time. Dr. Burman following my eyes with his.

"Okay," he said. "Why don't we break a little early. You've done some good work in here today, Jenniffer."

"I have? How do you figure that? It feels like it's always the same conversation with you and nothing changes."

"You do have feelings. See. You just acknowledged it. You are not as dead and as numb inside as you think. You are starting to open up a little for one, and that itself is a huge step. It let's me know that you are starting to trust in me and the work we are doing here; even if you don't feel that yourself as of yet."

Dragging my pole back up to my room, I wondered how much of what Dr. Burman had just said was the truth. *Was I actually starting to trust him, and why did I go and blab and tell him about the numbers in my head?* Counting the steps as I climbed up the stairs, I regretted confiding in him already.

28

Ameliah was sitting at the foot of her bed when I finally returned to our room. A small gray overnight bag with the words Long Jet Airlines stamped in bold navy print was on the bed next to her.

"You're not leaving today, are you?" I asked her nervously.

"Why don't you tell me," she said with a snarky tone. "You're the one who read the charts aren't you?"

"Yes, but ...."

"But what?"

"But ..... but..... well," I paused not really sure what to say. "You just shouldn't answer somebody's question with another question, that's what." I remarked cheekily.

At the same moment we both started to laugh, and for the first time in days, Ameliah's smile actually looked genuine for a brief moment. Then just as quickly it diminished, and I sat down beside her.

"I don't want you to leave here being mad at me," I said bumping shoulders with her. "You're my only friend."

"I'm not mad at you."

"Yes you are."

"No. I'm really not."

"Well you were."

"It wasn't that I was really mad at you Jenniffer. It was more like the fact of you knowing what my chart said made it all too real all of a sudden. Like until someone else knew, it was all a dream and once you knew the truth, I had to wake up. I can't hide anymore, you see. It forces me now to face things."

"Face what things?"

"This," she said pointing to her bag. "That it's time to leave here for good soon."

"But I thought that's what you wanted, what you've compromised your values in this place for?"

"To a point."

"So why do you seem like getting out of here is suddenly at the bottom of your list?"

"It's not that easy out there for me Jenniffer. I have all these pressures and rules I'm forced to abide by."

"But they're not anyone else's rules, they're your own."

"No, that's just it. They're not. They're my fathers. They're my mothers. They're the airlines. I have more freedom in here than I ever will out there it seems."

Ameliah stood up and swung her bag over her shoulder.

"I should get going," she said solemnly. "My parents want me to meet them in the lobby at precisely fourteen hundred hours."

"You will be back to visit me though, right? You'll keep in touch?"

"Oh I'm not leaving for good yet. I am just going for tonight. I'll be back tomorrow afternoon sometime."

"So you're not being discharged today then?"

"Not officially for a couple weeks. This is just my first orientation back into the 'real world' as they like to call it. There are four altogether, so you are stuck with me for a few days yet."

"Well good," I smiled. "All the same, I'm going to be so lost here without you tonight."

"You'll be just fine," she said straightening her posture, then giving me a salute. "Until tomorrow afternoon my friend."

I laughed again, but she didn't crack even a hint of a smile this time. She just turned robotic like, and departed like an obedient soldier.

Later that night I was jarred from my sleep by the constant, low frequency ringing of telephone at Ameliah's vacant bedside.

"Jenniffer? Jenniffer, is that you?"

"Uh huh," I croaked, still half asleep, finally dragging myself up to answer it. "Who's this?"

"It's me, Ameliah. Thank God you heard my phone ringing and answered it."

"Well it's been ringing off and on for twenty minutes now you know."

"I know, and I'm really sorry, but I really needed to talk to you, and with you on restriction and everything, this is the only way I could think of to get a hold of you."

"You're not mad that I woke you, are you?"

"No." I yawned.

"I'm so glad you finally answered. Be careful not to get caught though, okay. I don't want to get you into any more trouble."

"Don't worry about me," I yawned again. "What time is it anyway?"

"O three hundred hours."

"Where are you?" I asked rubbing my eyes, trying to bring my surroundings into focus in the dark.

"Still at my parents house."

"Okay, so why are you calling me?"

"I needed to talk to someone I could trust, you know, someone who understands?"

"Ameliah, are you crying?" I was suddenly wide awake with concern. The line was silent, except for a faint breathing sound on the other end, so I knew we hadn't been disconnected, and the line was still open.

"Ameliah? Are you still there? It sounds like you are crying. Are you okay?"

"No."

"Talk to me Ameliah. What's wrong?"

"No, I'm not okay, and I am afraid I never will be," she cried. "I just don't think I can do this anymore Jenniffer."

"Do what?"

"Any of this. You know, play this game. Keep up this charade. I'm just never going to be good enough," she sobbed. "Nothing I ever do will be good enough, and I don't think I can go on anymore pretending it will be. That I will be."

"That's nonsense. Good enough for who?"

"My parents, friends, family, coworkers. Anybody. Everybody."

"You're good enough for me. Too good of a person and friend for me even."

"Oh please. I've been treating you like crap lately, and don't try and deny it."

"I will so deny it! Sure, you've been a little moody at times maybe, but who hasn't been?"

"Moody? Right. That's an understatement."

"Don't be so hard on yourself. You'll do nothing more than drive yourself crazy that way."

"Look who's talking."

"Exactly! And God knows we don't need two of me running around."

"Well better than two of me. Better than even one of me."

"Come on Ameliah, don't say things like that okay. You are an amazing woman and one of the kindest, most gracious people I know. Even if you don't feel like it at this moment, deep down you must know it's true."

"Not good enough though. I'll never be good enough."

"Stop being so hard on yourself. Nobody's perfect."

"You don't get it though, I should be. I should at least be closer to the top of the pile than I am. I should know better, but here I am still drowning in the bottom of the slush pile."

"Ameliah, hold on," I whispered. "I think I hear someone coming."

I managed to slip the receiver under the covers right before Catherine peeked into the room shining her flashlight.

"Jenniffer?" She asked. "Why aren't you in your own bed?"

"Um, uh, Ameliah's mattress is softer," I blurted. "Yeah, I uh, didn't think she'd mind since she is away for the night and all."

"Well I think you should get back into the bed that is assigned to you, and get some sleep. Alarms are only a few hours away, and I am expecting you to be where you are scheduled and should be, now and again in the morning."

After Catherine shut the door, I waited until I'd counted her walk fourteen steps away before I untucked the receiver.

"That was close," I whispered into the phone.

"Too close," said Ameliah. "You'd better go and do what she said before she comes back. You know she will check again."

"Yeah, I guess. Are you going to be alright?"

"I'll survive. Thanks again for picking up the phone. I do feel a little better than I did before I called, less anxious anyway."

"We'll talk more tomorrow when you get back okay. Until then, don't you believe anything negative about yourself, that means listening to your own self talk too."

"I'll try, and you don't worry about my bed either. I'll remake it myself when I get back."

"Such thoughtfulness and consideration from such a bad person." I teased.

"Ha, ha. Thanks again Jenniffer. I'll see you tomorrow okay."

"Anytime friend. Anytime."

29

I waited anxiously all the next day for Ameliah's return. She had been away just over twenty four hours, and it already felt like an eternity. When I got back to our room after finishing my chores that night, I was overly excited to see her sitting at her desk.

"You're back!"

"About twenty minutes ago."

"I thought you were going to be back earlier this afternoon, before supper."

"I was supposed to be, but you know how it goes."

"Sure do," I said diving onto her bed. "So, how are you feeling, better than last night I gather?"

Ameliah looked over at me squinting her eyes and crinkling her forehead.

"You're starting to sound like Dr. Burman," she said. Then she turned back to her desk, scribbled something rapidly across a paper, and lowered her voice saying, "And how are we feeling this evening Jenniffer?"

We laughed so hard that our eyes started to water, and both our guts ached.

"Hey," she said wiping her eyes, "You got your iv out, or should I even ask?"

"Or did I take it out myself you mean?"

"Well?"

"No, I got it out after lunch. I had to sign a contract with Catherine, Dr. Shaw, and Dr. Burman that I would drink a minimum of twelve hundred cc's a day if they took it out. I need to reach seven hundred and fifty calories to get this one out, and gain another four pounds," I said pointing to my nose.

"I'm gone for one day, and you're already making deals with the devil," she laughed. "I told you that you'd break."

"Ameliah," I asked in a more serious tone. "Are you okay? You were so sad last night when you called. What made you so upset?"

"It was nothing, really. Just the stress of being home I guess."

"I've never heard you like that before. You were crying and sounded so shaky. I didn't know what to say?"

"Yes you did, and you were right. It was just a weak moment, and I was over-thinking everything too much. It's over now, and I'm fine."

"Well I still think there is more to it, but if you don't want to talk about it now, I am here when you're ready."

"I know, and I thank you for that. You are a good friend Jenniffer."

"So are you," I said. "It's going to be so strange when you leave. You will have to secretly call me all the time, if I don't get my phone privileges by then."

"Two weeks? You will by then, I'm sure. And then you can call me anytime as well."

"And I will too. You can count on that."

"Good," she said. "Now if you could get over to your own bed, I am going to go have a shower and sleep in mine while I still can."

I got up and embraced her in a tight hug. "It's all yours roomy. It's good to have you back."

Before going to bed I picked up the journal Dr. Burman had given me at our first session and flipped through the pages. They were all still blank. I thought about what he had said about there being no rules when writing, and that the objective was to just get my feelings and thoughts out to gain a newly heightened perspective and awareness. I was still holding, staring at the open blank pages when Ameliah came out of the bathroom wrapping her hair in a towel.

"Hey are you writing?" She asked.

"Nope. Drawing a blank in my mind and on paper," I replied. "I understand how the process could be beneficial, but I just can't seem to format the things in my mind to words on paper."

"Did you get the, 'it doesn't have to be perfect, there are no rules' speech yet?"

"Almost every session."

"Yeah that was the tough part for me too. I was always afraid of how someone would judge or interpret my words if they ever read my journal. Then one day I guess I was so angry and frustrated with things, I just didn't care and started scribbling things down."

"I've seen you. You write every day, don't you?"

"Sometimes more than once. I have a small book in my purse that I keep with me all the time now, and write in it a lot too."

"So you really find it 'a helpful tool' as they call it here?"

"Pen and paper don't judge. You can write anything down as if confiding in a trusted friend, and you know it's safe."

"Has anyone ever read what you have written?"

"No. I've discussed some of the issues and feelings written about while in therapy, and I may have actually read some excerpts during, but no-one has ever actually read my journal."

"Why does Dr. Burman insist I take it to every session if he isn't going to make me read it to him then?"

"Oh that? Sometimes he asks me to review my most recent entries and we explore the feelings around them, but he's never asked to read it himself. You don't have to give him your journal and show it to him like homework he needs to mark if that is what you're worried about."

Ameliah brushed out her hair, and turned out her light.

"I'm going to the lounge to play backgammon with Penny for an hour before bed. We'll chat more later okay," and she was gone again.

Instead of waiting up for her, I put my empty journal back in my drawer and shut out my bedside light also. Not getting a good sleep the night before had left me exhausted all day so I crawled back into bed and drifted right to sleep.

30

The next couple of weeks were filled with continued compromise and acceptance on my end, which translated to cooperation and progress on paper. I'd been here at Caitlynne's Place now for over a month, and although I wasn't being defiant and objective any longer, I was still a long way from being released and going home. Ameliah however was going home tomorrow. I had been working hard to gain and keep my telephone, and in house privileges, but yet had been free to go outside other than to do my garden chores. Ameliah had kept in contact on her final three home visits, and we chatted for a good two hours on each one nightly. It reminded me of the nightly talks Steffi and I used to have, and how much I missed them. Every day since getting my telephone privileges I must have picked up the receiver at least once with the intention to call my sister, but always lost my courage. With her wedding being next month, I decided she probably didn't need me bothering her anyway, regardless what her weekly incoming letters said. Besides, my focus right now was on Ameliah, and as selfish as it was, how I myself was going to manage here without her. After a little get together socializing in the lounge downstairs to say her goodbyes to some of the others, Ameliah and I went back to our room for the last night so she could finish packing.

"How do you do it Ameliah?" I asked soberly. "You always seem to have the right answers for everything, and I'm not even sure of the questions."

"Ha!" She laughed. "I don't have all the answers. I just have an instinct for people. Give them what they want, tell them what they want to hear, and they'll eventually leave you alone."

"Well I sure wish I had your strength."

"It's not strength Jenniffer. You know that. I just do what I know is expected of me and play the game. You have all the strength. You're real. I'm just a better actress."

"Oh come on, that's not true and you know it."

"Look, for people like me, there is no winning. At anything. Leaving here for me isn't as big of a step forward as one may think. I'm not like you. For me making deals with the devil only takes me deeper down into the pits of hell. For people like you though, good people, it will help you find your wings so that you can gain your strength, fly up, and soar out of this pit to your freedom. My wings only carry me from one pit to the next."

"I wish you would stop saying things like that. They're simply not true."

"Things like what? That there's no hope left for me?"

"Precisely."

"There isn't. Not anymore."

"Well I don't believe that, and I don't think deep down you really believe that either. If there is hope for me, there is hope for anybody. You included."

I walked over to the foot of her bed where she was packing up her last bag and smoothed my hands over the sides of her comforter.

"Enough negativity. Did you notice my hospital corners? Because of losing our last bet it took me twenty minutes this morning to make your bed it did. Then it took twenty seconds to make my own." I admitted wittingly.

Ameliah turned away.

"Hey," I said, pulling her arm back around so she was again facing me. "Are you crying?"

She pulled and turned away from me again, obviously wiping her eyes, so I jumped in front of her.

"Talk to me will you. Tell me what's wrong."

"What you just said," she whimpered.

"About the hospital corners?"

"Precisely."

"Okay I'm confused. That was supposed to be funny and make you laugh not cry," I giggled. "Hey come on, I was joking!"

"I know you were, but others, they don't joke. You should have been there at my last home visit the other night. I'm so glad you weren't, but if you were, you would definitely get where these stupid tears are coming from. Where I come from, and am now going back to."

"I don't understand. Did something happen?"

"Same thing that always happens. I let everyone down. I'm an embarrassment to the family name, not to mention the woman I was named after."

She turned toward me with a haunting stare, tears streaming down her face like a faucet was opened behind her eyes.

"Sometimes I think it would be easier for everyone if I too just disappeared like Amelia Earheart did. If I just fell off the face of the earth somewhere, and vanished into thin air. Then at least my parents could say I lived up to her legacy right? I bet then they'd be proud of me."

I didn't know what to say. How could such a beautiful girl, with such a pure heart of gold and so full of life stand here before me, so empty of spirit inside that she wanted to disappear?

I leaned over, embracing her tightly in the circle of my arms.

"I'm sure that your parents are proud of you now Ameliah. I know my parents would be extremely proud if you were their daughter." I slid my arms back, clasping her hands in mine. "I'm proud of you too, and honoured to have you as my friend."

She squeezed my hands.

"Your friendship Jenniffer is the one thing I'm taking with me from this place that I will always cherish. I mean that too. It's funny how you can go through your whole life with people all around you telling you how much they love and care for you, and never feel it at all, isn't it? Then one day out of nowhere that one person comes along that never tells you they love you, but all you ever feel from them is love. Out of all the girls I have ever met in treatment and therapy over the years, you're the only one that I ever truly trusted. You're the only one that said she cared, that I know meant it; because I genuinely felt it."

"You make it sound like goodbye forever when you talk like that. We're still going to talk every night we can, and when I get out of here too, we'll still keep in touch. You know, just like the two women in that movie Beaches. The one with Bette Midler and Barbara Hershey. 'We'll be friends forever.'"

"I know the one. Friends forever."

"Well," I yawned. "I think I'll go climb into my own bed before Catherine comes in for checks and finds me on the wrong side of the room again."

I no sooner turned when the door opened, and we both laughed out loud as Catherine stepped in the room. She raised her eyebrows with curiosity, which made Ameliah and I laugh even harder.

"It's good to see you two girls in such good spirits," she said. "Don't stay up too late though. I know it's your last night together, which means you have a big day tomorrow Ameliah, and you need your rest too Jenniffer."

"I was just heading to bed when you came in," I said.

"And I'm going to finish some journaling, and run a quick tub before bed," said Ameliah.

"Okay. Well you girls have a good night then, and I'll see you both in the morning."

After Catherine left, Ameliah moved all her bags to the closet floor, and smoothed flat the comforter over her bed where they had all been.

"Do you need anything in the bathroom before I run my tub?" She asked.

"No, go ahead. Relax as long as you like. I think I'll be asleep as soon as my head hits the pillow. I'm beat."

"Okay, thanks. Hey, by the way, have you started journaling at all yourself yet?"

"Nope. Still nothing. I've picked up the book too many times to count now, but I never know what to write so I always put it back in my drawer. Are you going to keep writing when you get home?"

"This book will be finished after writing tonight."

"Wow. Again I haven't started and you're finished another book. What do you find to write so much about?"

"Poetry mainly. Sometimes I rant I guess, but mostly it's just random words that somehow eventually turn into verse of some form."

"I bet you've written some good ones."

"Do you want to read it?"

"Really? But it's so personal. You said nobody has ever read it."

"Of course you can read it. It's really nothing special though, so don't expect much."

"I'll be the judge of that. Coming from you though, it's probably good enough for publishing. Maybe it will inspire me to finally write something too."

"Nah, it's gibberish mostly, but you can read it if you really want to. I'll leave it for you when I'm finished writing tonight."

I switched off my light, and pulled my blankets up to my chin.

"Thanks," I said. "You're the best."

"Hey Jenniffer," Ameliah whispered through the darkened room, "For the record, I'm proud to have been your friend too."

31

It was just before six the following morning when I raced down the stairs to the Shaws' room, unaware that was where I was even headed when I started to run. I couldn't tell you how long I stood there before the door opened, if I had knocked, or if so, for how long. All I knew for sure was that Dr. Shaw was standing in front of me in his robe, and Catherine was somewhere behind him. I knew that he was saying something because I could see his lips moving, most likely asking me what I so desperately needed, but I couldn't hear anything. In that moment, the entire world as I knew it, stood completely still.

"Jenniffer?" Catherine's high pitched voice finally cut in breaking my trance. "Are you all right? Jenniffer? You look absolutely white, as if you've just seen a ghost?"

I still couldn't speak. In my mind I was screaming uncontrollable, ear piercing screams, but I was the only one who could hear them. My voice was stopped short at the back of my throat, my screams lost in transit.

"Jenniffer? What is it? What's wrong?"

Catherine's soft warm hands on my shoulders broke through my frozen stance, and I managed to turn my face toward the stairs. Then I collapsed in her arms, still looking upstairs towards the bedrooms.

"I'll go and check on things upstairs," I foggily heard Brian tell Catherine, after helping her lead me to sit down. Catherine pulled a woolen blanket from the closet, and wrapped it around my shoulders, supporting it with her arm around my back.

"Whatever it is Jenniffer," she said soothingly. "Don't you worry. I'm sure Brian will take care of it for you."

I shook my head ever so slightly, more in opposition of believing what I'd just seen, than in Catherine's attempts at reassurances.

"My husband is a very resourceful man, so I'm sure he can fix whatever it is that has you so distraught this morning. Things will be okay again in no time. Don't you worry," she tried to reassure me.

We both looked up when Dr. Shaw re-entered their room, shutting the door behind him when he stepped in. For a brief second, I held his wet eyed glance before following it to Catherine.

"What?" She asked now showing signs of deep concern. "Can't you fix it?"

"He can't fix this," I said in a dry whisper. "Nobody can."

Catherine stared at Brian as he knelt down before us, taking her left, and my right hand gently into his.

"I'm so sorry Jenniffer," he said sombrely. "I don't know what more I can say at this time other than that. I'm so very sorry."

"Brian?" Catherine demanded, with a quiver in her voice. "Will someone please tell me what's going on?"

"It's Ameliah, honey. She's gone."

Catherine shook her head.

"What? No, no, she can't be gone. There must some mistake. She's got to be here somewhere. It's not like Ameliah to just take off and run away. Someone should go check the pond. She's probably back there."

"No honey, she's not missing. I mean she's gone. I'd say sometime between two and three this morning."

"You mean she is .... ?"

Brian nodded.

"I'm presuming overdose. It appears she may have even had a change of heart shortly afterward though, and tried to purge whatever it was she ingested. There was just too much absorption by that time to amend it."

"I checked on her just after eleven last night, and she was laughing and smiling. Both her and Jenniffer were .... " Catherine stopped abruptly, and turned to me. "She said she was going to have a bath before bed, and you.... you were already heading to your bed when I said goodnight and left?"

"I woke up and went in to use the bathroom," I said, hardly parting my lips. "I didn't think to look and see if she was in her bed first, I just opened the door and walked in."

"Oh Jenniffer, you found her ..."

"I ....I just needed to use the bathroom," I said.

Then I collapsed.

32

The halls were eerily quiet later that day when everyone was finally allowed to set foot back onto the second floor. Not the kind of peaceful quiet when you are all alone, but the kind of quiet when the space you're in is shared with many people, all seemingly cloaked under a silencing spell, turned mute. I didn't have to make eye contact with anyone to be aware of at least a dozen sets of eyes now following my every step like a pack of hungry wolves eyeing their prey on a moonlit night. When finally reaching my room, I hesitated for a moment outside, then pushed on the door handle slowly, and slipped inside letting the door click shut behind me. I made my way over to my bed, and sat down mindlessly closing my eyes taking in a slow deep breath. Had the last few weeks, the last few hours all been part of a bad dream? Were all of my surroundings a hallucination or something I had conjured in my own mind?

Looking around the room, if one didn't know any different, that is surely what they would think. The door to the bathroom was now wide open, and the florescent white lights streaked newly polished stainless steel inside like tinsel on an overly decorated Christmas tree with snow white terrycloth towels hanging neatly over the bars. An unopened box of tissues had been placed beside a stack of new paper cups, and an unwrapped roll of toilet tissue hung over a newly lined waste basket. In the centre of the glossy tiled floor where I had found my best friends lifeless body only hours before, stood a bright yellow 'slippery when wet' caution sign. Ameliah's bed had been stripped of its sheets, and empty hangers that yesterday housed brightly coloured shirts and sweaters, now all pushed to one side, swung barren in the dark closet. It was if someone had come in with a mop and bucket, and washed away my only friends entire existence. It was no longer our room, but my room. Again I was left alone with that impending question that no-one could, or was willing to answer; why? I jumped up and bolted angrily across the room in search of some kind of clue. There had to be something, anything that would help me to understand why Ameliah had done this, and help me to be able to go on without her.

When I didn't show up in the dining room, Catherine of course came looking for me. I could see by the look on her face when she walked in my room, that she was somewhat nervous since not getting a response to her knocking. *What? Did she honestly think I was going to kill myself too,* I wondered looking back to the floor. I was sitting in the middle of the room, surrounded by an array of clothes, books, and miscellaneous items strewn around me. Every drawer and cupboard was empty and left ajar. Every shelf was vacant.

"Jenniffer, what on earth are you doing honey?" She asked, confused, I'm sure by the turmoil.

I tossed the book I had in my hand behind me, and grabbed another. I turned it upside down and flipped through the pages.

"I'm looking for something."

"So it appears. However, you were supposed to be in the dining room ten minutes ago. Did you not hear the bell?"

"So was Ameliah," I muttered under my breath.

Catherine hesitated to leave until I no longer acknowledged her presence any further, but went about my own business as if she had already left. A few minutes after she finally did leave, there was another knock on the door, and Amy, the housekeeper and recreation coordinator, walked in carrying a full dinner tray with an extra cup of coffee.

"Hi Jenniffer," she greeted me softheartedly.

I hadn't really made the effort to get to know Amy outside of the yoga and indoor recreational activities I was able to participate in, and I was in no mood now to make a new friend now.

"They've made an exception for you to eat in your room tonight, given the circumstances and the day you've had." She set the tray on my desk. "I've been asked to stay with you while you eat, and supervise though. You understand why right?"

"I'm not hungry," I declared.

Amy pulled back the drape to let the remaining sunlight of the day into the room, and sat down, cross legged on the floor beside me.

"If you tell me what it is you are so avidly searching for, maybe I can help you find it."

"I don't think so."

"Well maybe ...."

"Look, I don't even know what it is I'm looking for myself!" I yelled. "So there is no way you can help me! Okay?"

"Then how will you know if you find it?"

"I'll just know."

I scattered the pages of an emptied, loose leaf binder around the floor beside me.

"She wouldn't have done this without leaving me something," I mumbled. "Not me. I just know she wouldn't have."

"Who wouldn't have? You mean Ameliah? You think she left you something?"

"Well of course I mean Ameliah!" I snapped turning my head, staring coldly into her eyes. "I didn't mean the tooth fairy!"

Amy didn't flinch at my sudden attack, but held my gaze with an understanding eye.

"I'm sorry Amy," I said. "You didn't deserve that. I'm just, it's just that, oh I don't know." I turned my head to hide my sudden flow of tears. "I don't know anything right now, except that I'm so confused by everything. By all of this."

"It's okay Jenniffer. You don't have to be brave with me. Really." She leaned in towards me. "I understand completely what you're going through."

"No you don't! You don't understand at all what I'm feeling right now!" I shouted. "All of you people here go on and on saying the same stupid things over and over again like some old vinyl record skipping on a worn out turntable. You know why we're sick, why we all do what we do, and how you're all going to make the rest of us better. But you don't know, and you're not going to fix us all like you think you can! You can't! You don't have the slightest clue and you never will. That's why good people like Ameliah, the only person that really cared enough about me to want to understand me, had to keep coming back to this place." I looked into the bathroom, and then back to Amy.

"And now she is gone," I cried harder. "And all of you still go on pretending like you care so much. So much that in less than one day you come in and erase all that she was, like some simple mistake on an elementary school chalkboard."

Behind the tears I could see pooling in Amy's dark brown eyes, there was something that made me for some reason want to take back everything I had just said. It was something I had only seen before in Ameliah's eyes when we had shared our deepest feelings. There was an empathetic awareness that made me feel like, for some reason maybe, Amy really did understand.

"Jenniffer," she said with a steady voice. "You may be right in a lot of what you just said. I don't know what it is like to suffer the torment of an eating disorder, or how bad it must feel for someone to hate oneself so much that they are compelled to cut into their own flesh, and I admit neither does any of the other staff that I know of. What I can tell you though, is that we all do care very deeply for each and every one of you. You have to realize too, that you are each at your own stages of recovery here, and we work very hard to understand and accommodate each of you accordingly."

"Well if that's so true, then why the hell couldn't any of you help Ameliah? And what makes you so sure you can help me?" I cried.

"Because we all know how strong you are Jenniffer."

"Ameliah was strong. She was the strongest person I knew."

"She was a very strong young woman. She made her own choice though Jenniffer, and I don't think that once her mind was made up, there was anything that any of us could have done or said to change it. You Jenniffer can still choose to fight. And to live."

"But I don't think I have the strength to do this without her."

"You do. You might not feel it yet, but you do. You just have to keep fighting, and we'll all keep fighting right along side with you. One step, one moment, one hurdle at a time. Whatever it takes to triumph over this disease and win. You can do it."

"But I just want my friend back. I want Ameliah."

We sat silent for awhile, and then Amy stood up. I thought she was finally going to leave, but then she sat down on my desk chair.

"You couldn't know this Jenniffer," she said picking up a cup of coffee off the tray. "But from a personal standpoint, Ameliah's untimely death was very difficult news for me to hear this morning also."

"How so? I know she's talked about you before, doing the classes and all, but I wasn't aware you two were that close?"

"We weren't. Just over three years ago now though, someone who was very dear to me, as Ameliah was to you, took their own life also. And like you, I too was the one who found them."

"Really? Who was that?"

"Well if you'll get up and have something to eat with me here, I'll tell you," she said trying to force a ready smile.

"I'll sit with you, but I'm really not hungry. I don't think I can eat anything right now."

"Well at least you can try. If you can't finish everything on your tray, at least I can tell the Shaws' you made a valiant effort. You just got your last tube out, and I don't think Ameliah would want her death to be the reason you had to have it put back in again, right?"

I climbed up onto my bed and took the other cup full of hot water, unwrapped and dropped in a tea bag while glancing over the tray. The thought of any food, made my stomach churn.

"I honestly don't think that I can eat anything, Amy. Honestly. It's not an excuse to try and get away with abstaining this time either. My stomach is just so sick with emotion right now, I don't think I could really keep anything down."

She studied me for a few seconds, and then nodded.

"Okay Jenniffer, I believe you. I'd like you to put some milk and honey in your tea though. At least it's something."

I opened the 280ml carton of 2% milk, and poured some into my cup without measuring it. It wasn't that I didn't care if it was exactly two teaspoons I poured, I just didn't have the energy or the strength left to make the effort.

"So how did they do it?" I asked her. "Your friend I mean."

"He was a little more than my friend Jenniffer. Actually, he was my husband."

"What?" I asked shocked, looking to Amy's left hand. "But you're not wearing a ring?"

"I'm not married anymore."

"Oh my gosh," I said embarrassed. "I can't believe I just said that. I'm sorry Amy. That was really thoughtless of me, wasn't it?"

"No, it wasn't thoughtless. It was observant. It took me the better part of two years before I could finally muster the strength to remove my rings, and admit to myself it was really over. I actually took them off the morning I moved out of the house that we had shared together, and moved into here. It was an extremely difficult time for me, accepting the fact that he was really gone, and never coming back home. Sometimes even now when it's really quiet and I'm feeling lonely, I still want to deny it, and try to convince myself that he's just away on an extended business trip, and I will see him again soon."

"When I first came back into our room this afternoon, I tried to picture Ameliah like that too. Like she'd actually just taken her bags and gone home like she was supposed to have. That I couldn't call her because she was already back at work and already up happily flying over the South Pacific somewhere."

"Well I don't know how healthy it is to pretend and think like that, but it sure does help still to get me through some of the rougher days."

"Then the reality hits me too though, and I remember that Ameliah actually hated flying. Did you know that?"

"No. I didn't know that about her."

"Yeah, she was probably the best flight attendant in the history of aviation, and she absolutely hated flying." I took a sip of my tea, and put my cup back on the tray. "Amy, do you ever get angry at your husband for doing what he did?"

"Oh you bet. Sometimes I do."

"Part of me is so mad at Ameliah because she didn't even give me the chance to say goodbye to her. It almost feels as if she abandoned our friendship. Like maybe our friendship didn't matter to her the way I thought it did. Like it was all a part of her act. Then I get so angry at myself for even questioning her at all, and that maybe if I had just been a better friend, I could have helped her."

"It wasn't your fault Jenniffer. It's natural in situations like this to want to place blame, but you can't."

"But I knew Amy! I knew something was terribly wrong for awhile now, and I didn't do anything to help her. I didn't say anything at all, and then last night when I went to bed I knew it. Somewhere deep down I think I really knew it, and I should have done or said something to help her and now it's too late," I sobbed. "I was right here in the same room and I could have maybe saved her but I didn't. I went to sleep instead and let her die."

"Jenniffer, it is not your fault."

"Well that's what it feels like."

"I know it does, and for awhile it probably will. You have to keep reminding yourself though that it was the illness that took her life from us, and there wasn't anything any of us could have done or said to prevent it. That includes you."

"But why?"

"I don't know if those answers will ever be clear. I do think however, that whatever their reasons, neither my husband nor Ameliah believed they would cause any pain by their actions, but rather put an end to all the pain and suffering."

"So when will the pain stop then?"

"I don't have an answer to that one either. Some people will tell you time heals all wounds, but I don't know. For me, I try to take comfort in believing that the love and friendship my husband and I had the time to share, isn't confined to the boundaries of the time given here, but extends far beyond, and that we will again in time be reunited on another realm. Time heals for me because it closes the gap between the here and there. So until that time when my husband and I can be together again, I made a conscious decision to live each day I am alive to its fullest. To give the best of him that is in me, and be as present as I can in the here and now, because I know that is what he would have wanted."

Amy reached across and wiped the tears from my chin.

"I'm sure that is what Ameliah would want from you too, right?"

I layed back and folded my comforter over top of me like a sleeping bag.

"The Ameliah I knew, would expect no less from me," I said in a whisper. Then I closed my burning, swollen eyes, and went to sleep.

33

When I woke, Catherine was standing next to my bed.

"Hi," she said smiling softly. "How are you feeling?"

"What time is it?"

"Ten thirty."

I looked to the window. The drapes had again been closed.

"At night?"

Catherine nodded, and I turned over on my pillow.

"I brought you an ensure. I'd like you to drink it now if you would for me please."

I closed my eyes so not to see Ameliah's empty bed. *Whatever you want*, I thought to myself, forcing my body upright. I wiped the crusted tears that had dried beneath my eyelids, and blinked them open enough to see. I held out my hand, palm up. *You're not actually going to drink that are you?* The voice in my head screamed out. *That's five hundred calories! I don't care*, I thought back. *It doesn't matter. What the hell do you mean it doesn't matter? Of course it matters.*

"I remembered that you liked strawberry yogurt," Catherine said passing me the bottle, "So I thought you might like the strawberry flavour the best."

I twisted off the cap, pulled up the tab robotic like, gulped down the sugary cream, and passed her back the empty bottle. *You did it? And just like that? My God, you really have lost it now, haven't you? Do you even realize what you've just done? Shut up. I don't care right now. Please just leave me alone. I just want to be left alone.* I laid back down.

"Can I go back to sleep now, please?"

"Of course," said Catherine tucking a warm blanket around me. "Don't hesitate to come down and knock on our door if you need anything throughout the night at anytime. Even if it is only just to talk, or have someone to listen. We're here for you Jenniffer if you need us, okay."

Catherine left, and I cried myself back to sleep.

I awoke again at midnight, my clothes and bedding soaked in sweat and tears, and this time Susan was standing at my bedside, pressing a cool cloth firmly against my forehead.

"Stay still," she whispered. "Penny went to get help."

I tried to get up, but I didn't have any strength. My body was numb and trembling from the damp cold of my wet clothing.

"You were screaming out in your sleep, and woke us up. Not an easy thing to do either, wake up Penny. That girl can sleep through anything, I swear I think she hits her snooze alarm at least a dozen times every morning. Drives me crazy. I think you scared her half to death with your screaming and all. When we came in you were crying and flailing around in your bed like something had possessed you in the dark, and she ran right back out like a rat fleeing a sinking ship."

I took in a deep breath, and almost choked myself on the dry air just as Brian and Catherine entered the room with Penny in tow.

Shivering uncontrollably, I layed as still as I could while Dr. Shaw took my blood pressure, and flashed bright lights in and out of my eyes. He said something to Catherine I didn't hear, and then took Penny and Susan out of the room. I heard the door click shut behind them.

"Let's get you out of these damp linens before you catch a worse chill," Catherine said, untangling me from my bed sheets. "Do you have some dry pyjamas in one of your drawers I can get for you?"

"Catherine," I rasped. "Am I dying?"

She took my hands in hers, and guided me off my bed and onto my chair.

"No honey, you're not dying. I promised you I would never let that happen, remember? You have your sisters wedding to attend soon, and a full life ahead of you."

"Then what's happening to me? Why ....?"

"Your body is in shock. Not surprising considering the shape it's in, and all you've been through these last couple days. But don't you worry. We're here now, and we're going to take good care of you."

She quickly remade my bed with fresh, dry sheets, then pulled open each of my dresser drawers until she found something dry, and suitable for me to wear.

"Here," she said, holding up a full length grey and white flannel nightgown. "Let's get you into this."

"My sister gave that to me last Christmas," I said, not knowing why. "I have slippers somewhere back at my apartment that match."

"Well it feels very soft and warm."

She pulled it over my head and shoulders, and helped me climb back up into my bed.

"Hey now," she said wiping my cheeks with thumbs. "No more tears tonight, okay."

"I'm not meaning to cry," I whispered. "The tears just won't stop coming. I don't know how to make them stop. I can't ...."

"It's okay Jenniffer. Shhhh. They will stop in time. I promise, everything is going to get better for you in time."

Then I did something completely unexpected by either of us. As if instinctively, I reached out and wrapped both my arms around Catherine's waist in a tight bear hug. It felt almost like in that moment she was my only life preserver, and I held to her securely as if to keep me from drowning in my own tears.

"I'm scared Catherine." I sobbed. "I feel so empty, and alone, and I'm so scared. I don't want to die."

She pulled back and looked directly into my eyes.

"You listen to me Jenniffer. You are not going to die," she stated matter of fact. "Do you hear me? Because we won't let you!"

"How is she doing?" Dr. Shaw asked, entering the room with a tray.

Catherine stood up and patted my knees without shifting her eyes from mine.

"She's doing fine now," she said. "A little shaky still, but she's a tough one. Tougher than she knows."

"Yes she is," he said continuing on, while taking my vitals again. "I've brought you a glass of juice here, and something else I want you to take for me Jenniffer."

"What is it?"

"It's a prescription Dr. Burman and I are starting you on, and we want you to take it now on a daily basis. Remember when we discussed this in my office as an option? Well I don't think we should leave it as an option for you anymore. Especially with all the recent developments and stresses you're having to endure. I believe it is now going to be a significant requirement in your recovery process."

I looked down at the two little beige pills bouncing around the bottom of the clear cup he passed me. *How ironic,* I thought. *That the very thing that had just killed my best friend, was now a requirement for my survival.*

Catherine passed me the glass of juice, which I took in my other hand.

"I think you will find that this will help you sleep better too Jenniffer. Relax you."

Oh yeah, right? Relax you? No it will make you lethargic, and lazy! Then they can continue to pump all their fatty calories into you while you do nothing but lay around gaining more and more fat. Five hundred calories before, and now another seventy in the apple juice they gave you to take some stupid pills with. Not to mention whatever else they've secretly mixed into it. Nice try guys. Ask for fresh water.

"Can I have water instead please?"

"Not this time."

I swallowed the pills, drank the juice, and passed the empty cups back to Catherine.

"You lay back and try to get a good nights sleep now Jenniffer," she said. "You should start to feel the effects of the medication in about twenty minutes or so. I'll check back in on you around then. Good night."

"Good night Jenniffer." Said Brian. I'll see you in the morning at weigh-ins."

I sunk back into my fresh scented warm blankets, counting their steps as the Shaws descended the stairs, and tried not to listen to the voice in my head screaming loudly, incessantly, calling me every name in the book.

You spineless coward! Since when do you give in so easily? They say no water, so you drop back another seventy calories like a drunkard at the bar with his shot of tequila. Hey stupid, that's like one sixth of a pound you just put on you know. You should at least be doing some sit ups or leg lifts or something to burn it off don't you think. Hey fat ass? Are you just going to lay there like a pig in her pen, and let them fatten you up while they laugh all the way to the bank at your expense? Hey come on, don't be such a pushover. We've come so far, you can't quit on me now. Fine, whatever, you sleep now then, but we'll have to work twice as hard when you get up in the morning just to make up for this inconceivable submission tonight.

I laid in the darkness without moving for what seemed like an eternity, waiting, longing for those little pills to take effect, hoping for more sooner than later. Unable to make out the hands on the wall clock, I reached across and switched on my desk lamp. Only ten minutes had passed. I don't know what prompted my next move, but I reached into my drawer and lifted out my blank journal. Before turning off my lamp, and sliding the book between my mattresses, drawn into a sound sleep; I wrote.

I sit
I stand
I lay

Spinning recklessly
stretching forth
reaching
Empty hands
Cold
Lost
Cloaked in black
Hungry
Blinded

Inhabiting darkness
Overwhelming silence
stirring fear within
Trapped
in a compound
Anger
Pain
Despair

I sit
I stand
I lay

34

Ameliah's funeral was held in the late morning four days following her death, at a cathedral in her parents home town. Although I was still on in-house restriction at Caitlynne's Place, the Shaw's allowed me and five other girls in the house to attend the service with them. Amy and the Andersons also attended, which provided enough room in both the vehicles for all of us. Karen, Valerie and I rode in Amy's car with her, while Penny, Susan, and Allison went with the Anderson's. Amy and I didn't really do a lot of talking, but I don't think we needed to. As difficult as I knew this was going to be for me, I knew also that it was going to be difficult for Amy too. We were going to have to be strong today for each other.

The ceremony itself was very formal with about three quarters of the guests all dressed in full flight, Long Jet uniforms. Ameliah's parents stood at the front of the church on either end of her casket throughout the entire service which I thought was peculiar, yet not near as strange as their behaviours. I never saw either of them once shed a single tear in the loss of their only daughter. Ameliah's mother however, seemed more concerned with how her makeup was holding up under the bright florescent church lights, and her father, he seemed more annoyed, as if from some embarrassment surrounding the cause of his daughter's death, or rather 'the situation at hand' as he put it. Can you believe that? Their only child was being lowered into a dark hole, six feet below the earth's surface, and when I heard one of the other guests ask Mr. Prescott how he and his wife were coping, he replied coldly, in a stately manner that they were 'dealing with the situation at hand.' Sadly, I was beginning to see a glimpse inside that part of Ameliah's world that she worked so hard to conceal. Seeing things from her side and point of view, sent a shiver down my spine, causing goose bumps to explode over my arms and legs; not resulting from the cool summer breeze, but from the cold emanating from her parents.

Looking through my eyes, Ameliah seemed to have the perfect life, full of love, excitement, and glamour. I had envisioned her moving away from Caitlynne's Place, having her perfect career, her perfect body, and her perfect home and family. Through her eyes though, it was all perfectly empty and materialistic. She probably didn't even think of her suicide as killing herself because she felt like she was already dead. These people, her supposed family, had indeed killed my friend long before this.

Isn't it funny, I thought, *how people see things in other people's lives that they want, but they can't recognize in themselves, that they already have. It's right there in front of them. It's all around them. Yet they just can't see it, like the forest from the trees.*

Through my eyes, my life seemed empty and unfulfilled. Stale with disappointment and failure to achieve any goals of my own. Ameliah, saw things differently though. She always told me how much she envied the warmth and heartfelt love and compassion she saw within my family. She'd tell me how she didn't ever need to meet them to know how great my family was, because the letters and calls Caitlynne's Place received daily from them validated it all. I'd then tell her how I used to feel like that too, but that things were different now. I'd tell her how wrong she was, and she would stick to her guns and tell me how I was just being stubborn, because I was still angry. I wish she were here now so that I could tell her I finally realized that she was right. Furious as I still was, behind all the hurt and rage, I had to admit I had as close to the perfect family as anyone ever could have. My parents both had tears in their eyes when they had to walk away from me and leave me at Caitlynne's Place. Neither Mr. or Mrs. Prescott cried even one single tear walking away from their daughter for the last time; forever.

Did that mean they didn't love her? I had to believe not, but rather that they just never learned how to show it, or to share it. After all, I couldn't believe for an instant that anyone could ever have known Ameliah for less than a minute, and not loved her.

I found a quiet spot under a tree which I knew Ameliah would have loved away from the crowd, and sat down. I closed my eyes and smiled for the first time in days as I pictured Ameliah in my mind, sitting at her desk writing in her journal, then brushing out her long thick hair in even strokes. I imagined her standing up, smoothing over her bed sheets, then pulling out all the stray hairs in her brush and rinsing it off under the hot water faucet before replacing it on the top left hand corner of her desk, exactly one inch from the top and both sides.

"Jenni?" A familiar voice broke into my daydream. I opened my eyes, and turned.

"Steffanni? Is that really you? My God, what, what are you doing here?"

"When mom called to check in on you Monday, Catherine told her what happened."

"But how did you know I was here?"

"Catherine."

"Mrs. Shaw, Catherine?"

"Yep," Steffanni said, sitting down on the grass beside me. "She didn't want you to have to go through this alone, and although she said that she couldn't allow us any extra time after necessarily to visit, it wasn't against any laws that she could think of that prevented me or anyone else to attend a public funeral service."

"Catherine? Mrs. Shaw said that?"

"Mm hmm."

"And she told you what time, and where we'd all be?"

"I didn't hear it from her," Steffanni said, bending her fingers airing in quotes.

"But you never even met my roommate before, so why did you come here?"

"Because I know you, and you're my big sister," she said almost knocking me down, nudging my shoulder. "I thought you could use a friend. Mom told me how close you and your roommate had become, how difficult this week has been for you, and we didn't want you to have to go through it all alone."

"How the hell would she know?"

"She only calls that place to check in on you and to see how you're doing at least like twenty times every day!"

"She does?"

"Well okay, maybe not that many, but she does call at least once every day. Don't act so shocked sis, she's really torn up you know. She's convinced that you are never going to forgive her and dad for doing what they did to you Jenni. Going secretly behind your back and all."

"Nobody calls me Jenni anymore, Steffi. I go by Jenniffer now."

"Since when?"

"Awhile now, I guess."

"Yeah well, whatever you want. It's your name. Anyhow, mom really believes that you are going to hate her forever you know."

"I don't hate her," I stressed, while tugging up a dandelion, then popping its yellow top off across the grass in front of us.

"Don't tell me," Steffanni said abruptly, while grabbing another dandelion, then doing the same thing. "Tell her. She knows you have phone privileges now, and she sits by the phone constantly hoping you will call you know."

I looked up at her trying to remember when the last time I'd really seen her was. *When did she, my little sister, get so big? I wondered. So grown up? And so smart?*

"I can do better than that," I said. This time nudging her, myself reaching for another dandelion, now laughing.

"Hey, hold on you .... you .... you .... Jenniffer, you," she mimicked, picking another dandelion of her own. "Okay. Ready?"

"Ready."

Our hands assumed their position, and we simultaneously spoke.

"Ready. Set. Go!"

Then both at once, we popped the heads off our dandelions in a race for distance, just like we had spent hours doing in the grass when we were kids.

"I win!" I howled, laughing loudly.

"No way!," she said. "Best two out of three?"

"Deal. But winner still has to make the Queen's crown, and you know I'll always be the Queen."

"We'll see about that."

And we did. I won again, so Steffanni had to collect all the dandelions we'd picked, and braid them into my championship crown. When finished, she placed it on top of my head, and gently pushed my brittle, straw like hair behind my ears.

"Jenniffer," she said no longer laughing, but earnestly. Please hurry up and get better. I miss you so much, and I need you back home."

I embraced her in a tight hug, that hurt my back so badly, I had to pull away.

"I'll be home soon," I tried to reassure her. "I promise."

"You have to be home for my wedding okay. You know I can't get married without you. I NEED to have you there with me."

The way she stressed the word need, made me question if something wasn't wrong, and I was afraid to suppress any intuitive feelings again, so I pried.

"You're not having any doubts about marrying Rick are you? Getting cold feet or anything?"

Steffanni paused momentarily before answering, which made me even a little more suspicious, but then she broke into her usual smile.

"Of course I'm not having doubts. Richard and I are fine. I just need to have my big sister at my side too, that's all."

"Are you sure there isn't something more going on that you're not telling me?"

"Everything is fine Jenni. Really. I mean Jenniffer," she laughed.

Although I still wasn't completely one hundred percent convinced, and I was sure there was something more to the story she wasn't telling me, our visit was cut short by Amy informing us that we would be leaving to go back to the house in ten minutes. I still wanted to say my final goodbye to Ameliah, so Steffani walked back with me to the plot before we parted, telling me to please call mom, and also to call her. When she was gone, I turned back toward the freshly disturbed soil of Ameliah's grave, and knelt down.

"That was Steffani," I said. I wish so much that you could have met her. You would have really liked her. I still can't believe she's really getting married next month. My little baby sister. Can you believe it?" I brushed the damp soil with my palm. "Oh Ameliah, I miss you so much. I just don't know how I am going to get through all of this without you. Who am I going to talk to that will understand me? God I wish you were here. I wish we could have met before all of this. Before we got sick, and before things got so messed up. Then maybe things would have worked out differently for us because we would have had each other to turn to instead of our alter egos." Amy honked the car horn, letting me know we had to leave, and I stood up. "I have to go now, but I will be back. I will never forget you my friend. Never. I promise you that."

The entire drive back to Caitlynne's Place after the funeral, I sat twisted in the back seat watching out the rear window at the world passing behind me. The road ahead of me to recovery was going to be a long and difficult one to journey, and there was still a big part of me that didn't yet know if I even wanted to take it. I didn't know anymore who Jenniffer Cynthia Lynne Klark was without my eating disorder. On the other hand, who really was I with it? I had so many questions without answers that just kept generating new questions, my head felt as if it could explode. I wanted to get better for Ameliah, for Steffani, my family, and also for myself. I wanted to be healthier, stronger and happy. I wanted to be in control of my own life again, which was the one thing I knew my eating disorder wouldn't let me have. I was slowly learning and understanding how it had control, and if I wanted my life back, I had to let it go. I also didn't want to be fat either though, and that is one thing my eating disorder could guarantee me protection from. My pros and cons list was still even, and I was equally torn between the two. As Amy drove up to the front door at Caitlynne's Place, I wished even more Ameliah was here. She would talk things out with me. She wouldn't judge me. She would listen to me. She would understand me. She would truly empathize with me, and she would surely help me decide what I should do.

After stepping out of the car back in the drive at Caitlynne's Place, my mind wandered back to the day my parent's left me here, and I hesitated for a moment and looked up. That is when I saw her. The silhouette of a girl standing behind the drape that curtained my bedroom window.

35

Sprinting past everyone back up to the second floor, I cracked open my door, and peered into the room gasping for breath, before stepping in. I don't know who or what I thought I saw, or was going to find, but the room was empty. As much as I wanted to see her, to find her there, waiting for me, I knew Ameliah was gone, and no matter how much I wished otherwise, or refused to accept it, she was never coming back.

"You idiot" I thought looking into my mirror. *"Now you're hallucinating too? Seeing ghosts, things that aren't real? That's good. Real good, you fool."* I took off the wilted dandelion crown feeling even more like an idiot for forgetting I was wearing it, and draped it over the corner of the mirror. Then I saw her again, this time in the reflection of my mirror standing only a few paces behind me. I quickly blinked, closed my eyes, and counted quickly to fourteen before reopening them. This time though, the image didn't disappear. When I spun around, the girl jumped back alarmed.

"Who the hell are you?" I snapped fiercely.

"I'm Cassidy. Are you Jenniffer?"

"Uh, yeah, and this is my room. So you're obviously in the wrong place." I pointed to the door. "So you can leave now."

The girl didn't move. She just stood in front of me with a blank look on her face similar to a foreign exchange student that didn't understand plain English.

"That meant get out!" I demanded, pointing again to the door.

"I would if I could!" The girl yelled back to me. Then she sat down on Ameliah's bed dropping her head to her hands bursting into tears. "I wish I could leave right now and never come back!"

I shook my head in disbelief. Just what the hell did this girl think she was doing? She couldn't sit there.

"Hey, hey you. Get up from there!" I shouted. "You get up off that bed right now!"

I had no sympathy for her tears, as her sobs grew louder. "Get the hell up!" I shouted while charging my way, full blast across the room. "That's Ameliah's bed! You can't sit there!"

When the girl still didn't move, I reached across and pulled the bed spread right out from under her with such a force, that she crumpled to the floor at my feet with it.

"You have no right!" I continued shouting at her, tugging at the blanket. "Just go, and get your skinny ass out of here right now! What the hell is wrong with you? Do you not understand English? This is not your room! You don't belong in here!"

"Jenniffer!" Dr. Shaw yelled, while running into the room with Catherine. When I ignored them, he grabbed both my arms and held them securely behind my back, which made me even more hysterical, kicking and screaming.

"Get that little bitch out of here right now, or let me go, so I can do it myself!" I squirmed.

Catherine helped the trembling girl to her feet, giving me a dirty look, and walked her out of the room.

"And you'll stay out if you know what is good for you too!" I yelled through the closed door.

"Okay Jenniffer, that's enough now," Dr. Shaw said, letting my arms drop to my sides. "You really need to calm down."

"Calm down? I come in here after burying my best friend and find some strange kid taking up Ameliah's space, sitting on her bed, and you? You tell me to calm down? You must be crazier than you think I am Doc."

"I know you've had an emotionally, oppressive morning Jenniffer, and getting a new roommate at this time isn't necessarily going to be an easy adjustment, but unfortunately this is the only bed we have available right now, and we need it."

"Oh, and you need it do you?"

"Yes, Jenniffer. We need it. This young girl needs it. We have a very lengthy waiting list for admissions here."

"Waiting list, shmating list. This is bullshit!"

Catherine re-entered the room, and I glared at her with the resentment of the devil himself.

"You could at least have told me," I growled. "Warned me."

Catherine didn't acknowledge me speaking to her, but passed her husband something that looked like a pen which she had cupped in her palm, and then they both stepped toward me.

"What?" I demanded. "What now?"

The last thing I remember of that day, before the room went black, was a sharp prick in my left shoulder, a warm tingly sensation flowing through my arm, and someone supporting my back. Then I was out.

36

In the darkness of my dreams I fought many demons. I battled one after the next trying desperately to reach the light in front of me that was fading quickly, which seemed so far out of my reach. When all had seemed lost and all hope was gone, I dropped to my knees, let go of my sword, and waited in the dark cold, ready to surrender to all that scared me most. Then suddenly the light I thought had gone out forever, began growing closer, and closer, eventually casting a warm bright glow over me. When I looked up, feeling bruised and broken, I looked upon the face of an angel. Ameliah was with me. I knew it was her by her spirit, and when our eyes met, she spoke to me without speaking.

"Up now Jenniffer," I heard her in an angelic voice. "You my friend are a fighter, not a coward. You are strong beyond your means, and you are not alone. I am still here with you, and haven't left your side. All you have to do is open your heart and look for me. Look inside and you will always find me there. Do not fear the dark my friend, you will always have my light to guide you when you need it to see. Now stand. Rise up and awake. Dry your tears and once more draw your sword. I will be your shield, and against this war, we will together claim a victory."

When I opened my eyes, the sun's rays were just breaking through the nights sky, and the birds were twittering about their morning routines in search of something to eat. Overwhelmed by my dreams, I decided again to try writing in my journal. This time though, when I reached my hand between my mattresses to retrieve it, I felt something more. Something I hadn't noticed before. I crawled out of bed, and lifted my mattress as high as I could. Behind my journal, pushed a little further back, lay another book. It was powder blue, with random abstract designs drawn over it with coloured pencils detailing both the front and back covers. I recognized it immediately. It was Ameliah's. I took the book and climbed back on top off my bed. I knew Ameliah wouldn't have left without leaving me something I thought, and I should have known if anything, this is what she would have left for me. I also should have known without giving it a second thought, that she would have left it there since that is the place she had always kept it, on her side. After tearing apart the entire room, between the mattresses, the place I should have known to look, was the one place I didn't search at all. I remembered back to the last time I saw Ameliah, and how we had discussed journaling. I remembered how she had told me that I could read her journal, and that she would leave it here for me later that night when she had finished her last and final entry. If only I'd known then that she really meant she was giving it to me as her way of saying goodbye, and something to remember her by. If I had only pried and pushed her a little more, maybe then I could have changed the outcome. Like a movie, I rewound and played the last conversation we had over and over again in my mind, and relived our last few moments together. Then I remembered her in my dream. Ameliah was indeed still with me in spirit, and she always would be. I clutched her journal tightly to my chest smiling, and breathed in deeply the scent of her lilac perfume that still lingered upon its paper. My shield.

37

When I heard the bathroom door click open, I turned.

"Oh. You again," I mumbled, still feeling slightly groggy from whatever was in the shot that Dr. Shaw had given me the day before.

"Sorry," the girl apologized in a cowardly fashion. "I didn't mean to bother you."

I glanced up at the clock, six twenty a.m., then back to her. She was so tiny. Not a short tiny either, but an unnatural tiny. A sickly, malnourished thin, like a twelve year old child that had been starved since the age of ten. I recalled my attack on her, and was amazed that she hadn't shattered when I knocked her off the bed to the floor like a glass china doll falling off a mantle. I knew I should have been somewhat embarrassed by my previous actions the day before, but while watching this girl move, I almost burst out laughing, realizing I must have scared the poor little thing half to death with all my screaming and lashing out. I had to give her a lot of credit for taking it though. On the outside she is tiny, but on the inside, this girl was as tough as nails. I wondered if she was scared to come back into our room, or fearful to sleep thinking I might attack her again, and try to kill her off or something while she slept in my dead roommates bed?

She moved around her side of the room stealthily and nervously as if afraid to sit down or touch anything, knowing I was now awake and watching her.

"No bother," I finally said.

She looked over with her eyes, only slightly turning her head.

"Pardon?" she squeaked dryly.

"I said you didn't bother me."

"Oh. Okay. Good."

I continued to watch her as she moved her tiny frame across the room to the door, and she reminded me of Jack trying to sneak away from the menacing giant, in the fairytale Jack in the Beanstalk.

"You said it was Cassidy, right?" I questioned loudly. "Your name?"

She nodded.

"Well Cassidy, come here for a minute will you?"

The girl stopped short in her tracks with her hand on the doorknob, like a jewel thief caught red handed in the night. Her entire body stiffened.

"I promise, I'm not going to hurt you," I said. My words seemed to put her somewhat slightly more at ease, but still I don't think she was convinced. "Look, I know I didn't exactly make a very good first impression yesterday, but the fact is, that we are going to be stuck in here together as roommates for awhile, and I think that warrants a second chance. Don't you? It's not like you have somewhere else to go to or have to be. Weigh-ins aren't for almost another half an hour yet, and I'm sure you're not that anxious to be there standing in the hall waiting."

She looked at the clock, shrugged her pointy shoulders, and walked over while still keeping a couple of feet, and an arms reach between herself and my bed.

"I really am sorry about yesterday," I apologized. "Even if it seems I don't really mean it. It's just that my last roommate, the girl that was in here before you, well it's hard for me accepting that she's gone, you know."

"I know. They kinda told me a little bit yesterday. She killed herself in this room, right? Creepy."

I glared up at her, and she almost fell backwards.

"SHE was my best friend," I said stressing the 'she', "and 'SHE' had a name. Ameliah."

"Um, I'm sorry for your loss," said Cassidy anxiously. "I didn't mean any disrespect. I just meant ...."

"Yeah I know what you meant. You and everyone else too. Anyhow, forget it." I extended my hand in an effort to make peace. Although I didn't like seeing this new girl anywhere near what was only a few days ago Ameliah's space, I also knew I didn't have a choice. I was going to have to learn to deal with it, and to make the best of it while I had to.

"I'm Jenniffer. Jenniffer Klark."

"Cassidy Mills," she said shaking my hand cautiously, then again stepping away.

"Here," I said straightening out my comforter. "Sit down and tell me all about yourself. From the looks of you, we're probably going to be roommates for a long time."

"What's that supposed to mean?" She asked a little less guarded, and with a little more attitude.

"Nothing," I smiled. "Let's just say you kind of remind me of someone else that's been stuck in here for awhile, and leave it at that."

And so she did. This guarded, defensive, emaciated shell of a girl sitting in front of me reminded me of someone I knew very well. She reminded me of me.

38

Before going downstairs for weigh-ins, through our brief conversation, I found out that Cassidy was a skater, with the ambition to go pro. At only fifteen, she had already won notable awards and trophies in various competitions throughout North America, and she definitely had her sights set high on an Olympic gold in her future. Looking her over, and listening to her speak, it was hard to see someone with such great ambition and drive, to be forced to take a time out due to this overpowering disease. At the same time though, it was hard to imagine how in her emaciated state that she actually had the strength needed in her spindly arms and legs to even lace up a pair of figure skates, let alone perform a triple sow cow. On one hand I felt sorry for her being stuck in here, and yet on the other hand, if I was to be completely honest with myself, I would have to admit, there was a part of me that was as green as a granny smith apple with envy. I burned with jealousy that she was able to achieve such a state of thinness.

After weigh-ins, and we were back in our room awaiting the breakfast bell, Cassidy started asking me questions about Susan. It seemed that Cassidy had been referred to Caitlynne's Place from Linwood County Hospital, where she had been an outpatient for the last year, and Linwood was the same hospital that Susan had also been transferred from to here. Cassidy said that she didn't think Susan recognized her from any of the hospitals group programs, and I told her that if she had, I was sure that Susan would be knocking on the door at any moment, followed of course, by Penny. It was no surprise to either of us, when exactly fifteen minutes before the breakfast bell sounded, Penny and Susan rapped on the door, and walked in.

"Hey lady," Susan shot out. "How are you feeling? You look like death warmed over."

Penny gave Susan a sharp jab in the arm with her elbow combined with a fierce scowl.

"Ow! What the heck was that for?"

Penny just glared at her.

"Oh. Um, sorry Jenniffer. I didn't mean to say death-"

I twisted myself around and took a quick look at my reflection in the mirror.

"Sorry for what? I do kind of look like death warmed over, don't I?" I said lightly. "I think it's these pills Dr. Shaw has been getting me to take at bedtime. They make me groggy. Hard to wake up and stay awake, you know." I yawned.

"Yeah, well you'll get used to that in time. So anyway," Susan said briskly, tipping her head toward the other side of the room. It was obvious she didn't come in just to collect me for breakfast. "Who's the new girl?"

"Her name is Cassidy something. Recognize her?"

Susan looked over, then shook her head.

"Don't think so. Why? Should I?"

"She just came from Linwood County somewhere. She was in their hospital's outpatient program, and thought she recognized you from there."

"Really? Hmm, well maybe. After awhile all the skinnies start to look the same I guess. Did you get the goods on her game?"

"Not completely. She's definitely a flusher and is pretty ticked that they searched her belongings and took away all her diuretics. She seems pretty confident that she won't be here very long either, and said that her mom will have her out before her next competition. She's some sort of hot shot figure skater or something. That's all I know.

"A skater you say?" Questioned Susan, looking more curious. "Come to mention it, I think I may have seen her before. If she's the one I'm thinking of, she attended this one group I was in that was held after clinic hours, but was open to both outpatients as well as inpatients. If it is her, her hair was longer then, and she only attended two groups before dropping out. No paperwork to hold her. She wasn't overly chatty, but she was always making sure she was the centre of attention, and had to be noticed. Good attention or bad, she didn't seem to care. As long as the focus was on or about her, it was all considered good."

"Well she didn't seem to have any reservations about going down to weigh-ins this morning, that's for sure."

"Probably scoping out her competition," Penny said sarcastically, which worried me a little. Penny had been doing really well lately curbing her obsession to compete with all of us to be the thinnest in the house, and I didn't want to see her comparing herself now to this new girl.

As the breakfast bell rang, the four of us made our way out of the room, and I watched as Penny hurriedly stepped into Cassidy's shadow, then glanced behind her to see if she had fit.

For Penny's sake, I was glad this girl was my roommate, and not hers, even if it did mean tolerating her taking up Ameliah's space. The voice in my head disagreed however, and fought me on this and everything else it could, over the next hour. The war going on in my mind was a true battle of wills between angel on one shoulder, and devil on the other.

Where's all this compassion coming from all of a sudden? And what for?

'I just don't want to see Penny self destructing again. That's all.'

Oh really? Well why do you care about so much about her all of a sudden anyway? You have more important things to worry about don't you think? Or don't you care anymore?

'It's not all of a sudden. I've always liked Penny. And Susan. They're my only other friends here now you know, except for Amy, but that's different. She understands things on a deeper level, and I can really talk to her at times.'

Amy now too? They're really suckering you in here, aren't they? They're brainwashing you, you know.

'Nobody's brainwashing me.'

Then why do you care so much about what they think? How they feel?

'What's so wrong with caring about someone else?'

Nothing, as long as you don't lose yourself in the process.

'I'm not losing myself.'

No? I think you already have. It's like you don't even care anymore.

'I care.'

Sure you do.

'I do so care.'

Okay, then prove it. How many calories did you just consume?

I looked down at my breakfast tray; three quarters of the way emptied, and began nervously twirling my stainless steel fork through my fingers like a small baton.

'Um, toast seventy two, milk one hundred and thirty, that's two hundred and two I think, and then some fruit salad, that's ....?'

Exactly the point. You don't even know, do you? You've just sat here shovelling the fat into yourself totally unaware. Then you'll go back upstairs and lay around moping, waiting for what? All the fat to blow you way up, that's what. You're slowly destroying all that we've accomplished, and don't bat an eyelash over it. Yet you're getting all worked up and worried about Penny self destructing? Yeah they're getting to you all right. They're winning because you are too weak to fight anymore for what you want. You're giving in!

'Well, I don't mean to .... I mean I don't want to .... I mean .... oh stop! Please just shut up and leave me alone. You're not real! You're just a voice in my head! You just don't understand!'

Oh contraire my dear lady, but I do. Look, it's all very simple. You have only four weeks until your sisters wedding right?

'Yeah.'

And how much do you weigh again now?

'I don't know.'

Aha you don't even know! So do you want to be fat or thin? Ugly or pretty?

'Not fair. You already know that I don't want to be fat and ugly anymore. And not just for the wedding either, but ever again!'

Really? Then why aren't you listening to me anymore? Why are you letting these people push you around and allowing them to make you fatter again. We only had a few more pounds to lose, and now we have no clue where we're at because you haven't been paying attention.

'Well I'm sorry, okay!'

No, not okay. Have you even looked in the mirror lately? I mean really looked at yourself?

'No. I guess I haven't. You know it' s discouraged here.'

Well you should. It's disgusting.

'You mean I'm disgusting'

Well? If the dress size fits.

'That's mean.'

No. Just true.

'Okay smart ass. So how am I supposed to fix that? I'll just always be disgusting then.'

Not if you start listening to me again you won't. You weren't disgusting when you got here were you? You were happy until then. Remember?

'But it's different in here. I can't control ....'

Can't? Or won't?

'Can't'.

Ha! Excuses!

'But ....'

But yes you can. We can. You just have to trust me again, that's all. I'll show you all the ways to get around the things they want you to do in here that we know will only hurt us, and before you know it, everything will be good again. Trust me.

When the bell rang signalling the end of breakfast, I set my three quarter emptied tray at the window, and followed Cassidy up the stairs. I was so confused. Part of me wanted to again listen to that voice in my head that had kept me safe for so long, and forget everyone and everything else. Then there was the other part of me that had been getting stronger again, and I didn't want to be a prisoner anymore either. To this place, or that voice.

Back in our room, Cassidy went to her side of the room without speaking, and I went to mine. I had fifteen minutes before rec class and I needed some real understanding and guidance. Last week at this time I would have just talked to Ameliah, so as an alternative, I did the next best thing. I pulled out her journal and read her final entry I knew in my heart she had written for me.

      A Simple Girl
      Once
      Strong as One
      Silent Now
      In a Struggle
      As Two
      Wasting Away
      Entangled
      Shackled
      In Chains
      Her Own
      Shadows

So Much
To Lose
Too Much
To Gain

Her Eyes
They Weep
Swollen Shut
In Sleep
In Darkness
There is Light
Beyond
New Life
She There
Can Breathe
She Is
Finally Free

39

"I found it," I told Amy after class.

"Found what?"

"What Ameliah left for me."

"Really? And?"

"She left me her journal."

"Wow. That's a really personal item. Are you sure she meant it for you, and it didn't just get left behind when they cleaned the room?"

"Oh yes, I am sure all right. One of the last things she said to me was that I could read it, and that it might help me to be able to start journaling myself. And after all that searching, you will never believe where I found it. It was right there under my mattress the entire time."

"Wow."

"Yeah. She used to keep it under her mattress when she was here. I don't know why I didn't think to look there first, but at least I am the one who found it, and not Catherine when she changed the sheets the other night."

"Well, have you read it yet?"

"I just found it this morning, but I did read her final entry."

"And? Did she write anything to shed new light on her intentions or why she did what she did?"

"Not exactly. But remember when you told me you didn't think there was anything I could have said or done to change her mind?" Amy nodded. "Well I think you are right. I could have possibly talked her out of it for awhile had I known that is what she was thinking about doing, but it would have only postponed it I think. It was like she was ready to go and she had her mind made up. She was at peace with it I think, as crazy as that sounds."

"Wow. I don't really know what to say?"

"There's nothing really to say I guess. I just thought I'd let you know after all that mess, I found it.

"Well I'm heading into town with Patricia now but we should be back by lunch. If you need or want to talk later, you know where to find me okay. Hey, are you going to tell Dr. Burman about Ameliah's journal?"

"I don't know. I didn't really think about that. I don't see him until tomorrow though. Why? Do you think I should?"

"Only if you want to. Ameliah left it for you right, not anyone else. If you want to share all of it or parts of it, that is completely up to you. You don't have to if you don't want to though."

"Ok, well there's the bell, so I better get going too. Chat later?"

"Like always, anytime."

My mind raced all day with questions about what to do with Ameliah's journal. I hadn't thought of sharing it, or giving it to anyone else until Amy mentioned it. *Should I tell Dr. Burman about it when I see him tomorrow afternoon? What about the Shaw's? Should I let Catherine see it? And what about Ameliah's parents even? Maybe I should give it to them? After all, she was their only child. But then again, Ameliah didn't leave photocopies for everyone or a note to pass it on, she left it only for me. She trusted only me with her words.* After a lot of thought, I decided for the time being at least, I would keep Ameliah's words silent for myself.

40

During my next few sessions with Dr. Burman, we didn't discuss how I was coping with Ameliah's death, or adjusting to having a new roommate. We focussed instead on ways of quieting the naysaying voice in my head, and curbing the time consuming rituals I had come to use as control and coping tools. This was not easy, and although he seemed to think we had a breakthrough in some way, I was not so sure. His theory was that as long as we kept open the lines of communication between us, and I continued to be forthright with him about these things, that this was a substantial step forward in my recovery. For me though, it seemed that the more I focussed on, and acknowledged these things, the more prevalent they became for me. The louder the voice in my head became, and the more ritualistic my routines and behaviours became. I just didn't get how giving so much attention to something negative, could be a good thing? "Acknowledgement and understanding," he would say, "are the keys to change." First, I had to acknowledge my behaviour. Secondly I had to explore the why's for the behaviour. Thirdly, I had to rebut the first two, and that was what was going to help me change and replace the negative thoughts and behaviours with positive ones. I was learning how to reprogram my mind like reprogramming a computer with a virus. My virus was my eating disorder, and it was not an easy fix. Dr. Burman gave me a workbook a couple weeks ago that I was to carry with me at all times, and every time I had a negative thought, he wanted me to write it down. I laughed at him joking that I would be doing nothing but writing consequently all the time doing nothing else, but he challenged me nonetheless. With every record I wrote on the left side of the page, I then had to write in the adjacent right hand column the opposing thought or feeling. I was a long way away from actually believing the positive, but I was however starting to challenge some of the negative, and I was beginning to feel a little more courageous and stronger again in my own right. Confronting myself was one thing, but conjuring the strength to face some others was a much more difficult task. With Steffanni's wedding now only one week away, I had to get out of my own head for awhile and think about her. I had to put everything aside and think about my family. It was time to swallow my pride and make some calls.

"Mom," I said nervously while gripping the receiver.

"Jenni?" She exclaimed, questioning my voice. "Jenni? Is that really you?"

"Yes, mom. It's me."

"Stu! Stuart come here! Come quick, it's Jenni! Stu, it's Jenni, she's on the phone!" My mom started screaming excitedly and crying. "Jenni, oh Jenni, I am so glad you called! I have been so hoping you would but, well, oh here's your father too. I am putting you on speaker okay. Here Stuart listen, it's Jenni!"

"Hi dad," I said trying not to both laugh and cry at my mother's outburst.

"Jenni, it is so good to hear from you honey. You must know your mother has been worried beyond sick. She's hasn't gone anywhere without her phone all summer."

"I'm sorry. I know I should have called before now but...."

"Oh never mind that now. We're just so happy to hear you." Mom sobbed. "Does this mean you forgive us Jenni? We're so sorry we had to lie to you and .... "

"Mom stop. Please. There is nothing to forgive. If anything, I am the one who needs your forgiveness. I did and said so many horrible things to you, and you didn't deserve any of it. I am the one who is sorry."

"I am relieved to hear you say that," my dad interjected. "You understand why we did what we did then? And I take it that you are doing better?"

"Yes dad, and I know it wasn't easy. I'm sorry you had to go to your friend and co-workers. I imagine it was pretty embarrassing for you and..."

"Nothing I do for my girls is embarrassing. I will do whatever I have to do to ensure their well being and safety, and I am damn proud of it too. As I am you."

"Thanks dad."

"You talk to your mother now, and we will see you on Saturday?"

"Yes dad. I will be there. The recreational director here is going to escort me."

"Good. It is going to be a big day. A good day."

"Yes it is." I could hear my dad whisper something to my mom, and give her a kiss on the cheek as she clicked off the speaker. One week from now and my baby sister was going to be a married woman. I could only hope she would be as happy as my parents were, and just as much in love in another forty years herself.

"Jenni, are you still on the line?" my mothers weepy voice cut into my thoughts.

"Yes, I am still here."

"I just wanted to tell you again how proud we are of you. Mrs. Shaw said that you signed a new contract with them, and that you have been cooperating and working really hard."

"I'm trying mom. It is really difficult, but I am trying. It's hard because I know I have gained weight, but I don't know how much."

"Maybe it is a good thing you don't know. There is a reason they don't tell you."

"I understand that. I'm scared what people are going to think on the weekend when they see me though. They are going to think I look..."

"Beautiful," she said cutting me off. "They are going to think you look beautiful."

"Thanks mom. What time are you and dad going to the church? I was hoping to get there a little early so we had time to maybe visit for a bit, with Steffanni too maybe?"

"We will be there by noon. Melinda is taking your sister to get her hair done, and then we will meet them at the church in the dressing room. Have you spoken with her yet? She was hoping you could be there early also."

"I called her last week, but not since then. I'm sorry again I didn't call you and dad before now too. Steffi said you were talking to Catherine on a daily basis, and knew I had phone privileges. I wasn't trying to hurt you, I just didn't have the courage to face you yet."

"Yes, I know. Steffanni told me that too. And I am sorry about your roommate honey. Ameliah, wasn't it? I so wanted to be there for you, but I thought it was better if I didn't force it."

"Probably right. Thanks for sending Steffi though. Anyhow, mom, I really should go okay. I have some laundry chores to finish tonight before lights out, and I need to get them done if I am going to be away Saturday."

"Of course, Jenni. I can hardly wait to see you. And hug you. If that is okay. Please say it is okay Jenni?"

"Of course mom, but only if you do one thing for me too?"

"Anything honey. Unless it means breaking any of your rules that is?"

"Just call me Jenniffer okay. I think I need to put Jenni behind me, and move forward with my new life now."

"Oh Jenniffer, you got it. That we can do."

"Thanks mom. I'll see you Saturday."

"Twelve o'clock. And Jenniffer, we love you."

"I love you too mom. Goodnight."

I hung up the phone with a smile. That call went better than I thought it would, I thought to myself. Then I went to finish my chores.

41

Friday night, before my sister's wedding, I was sitting back on my bed reading Ameliah's journal when Amy and Catherine walked in carrying a dress bag.

"Look what just arrived for you," Amy said enthusiastically. "Well, aren't you going to get up and go try it on for us?" She asked.

I slipped the journal behind me, noticing Catherine's quizzical look. I was pretty sure she recognized it as Ameliah's, but didn't say. Instead she took the dress bag from Amy, and hung it over a hook on the armoire unzipping it.

"Of course, she is going to try it on," Catherine chirped. "If it needs any touch-ups that way we have time to do them tonight."

I didn't move.

"Jenniffer, this dress is gorgeous!" Amy beamed.

I still didn't move.

"What's wrong?" Amy asked, sitting down beside me. "You look as if you've seen a ghost."

"Honestly?" I asked, looking to Catherine. "I'm scared. No. I am terrified."

Catherine pulled out my desk chair and sat down beside my bed.

"Okay. Talk to us," she said sternly.

"It's silly I guess. I'm being selfish. Tomorrow is about my sister, not me."

"Yes," Catherine agreed. "Tomorrow is about your sister. Tonight however is about you. So talk." She smiled and nodded. "Now."

"It's just that the last time I had that dress on, well, that is kind of where my life started to change. And not for the better. I never even thought about being overweight until I had that dress on, and someone thought I looked pregnant in it! My life spiralled out of control after that as you know, and I ended up here. I know I have been gaining weight again, and I'm afraid that dress is like a curse or something that if I put it on, I am going to spiral back again and I don't want to ruin Steffi's wedding being the fat, anorexic, or whatever, crazy sister."

"The only way you can ruin Steffani's wedding tomorrow Jenniffer, is by not showing up." Said Amy. "And I am going to be there with you the whole time too, remember? I won't let you do anything but have a good time, and take part in your sister's happiest day. I assure you."

"Promise?"

"Pinky swear," she said raising her pinky in the air.

"Exactly what Steffi herself would say to me if she were here too," I laughed, linking my pinky with hers.

"Okay, so it's settled then," Catherine said getting up and going to retrieve the dress. "The last time you had this on, you say it changed your life for the bad, right?"

"Yeah," I replied slowly and nervously.

"So the dress has been altered since then, and we could say that you have been altered too. I think you should go try it on, break any imaginary curse or doubts you have about it, and keep moving forward. What do you say?" She draped the dress over my arm, and motioned toward the bathroom. I looked to Amy, and she motioned the same also.

"All right, all right, I will try it on. Here goes nothing," I said hushed.

"Wrong," said Catherine loudly. "There does go something. Something very special."

"You!" Amy smiled pointing at me.

42

Amy and I arrived at the church the following morning at least half an hour before my parents or any other family, but the place was already bustling with activity. One of Steffani's sales staff that worked at the flower shop with her, saw me when I walked in, and ran over embracing me in a huge hug. She showed Amy and I to the dressing room, where we could wait, and I thanked her gratefully. This was my sister's day, I wanted it to be truly amazing and wonderful for her, and in the end it was.

The ceremony went precisely as Steffanni had planned, and all eyes were on her. Not even for a second when my sister entered the church hall accompanied by our father, did I myself even wonder where people were looking, or what they were thinking. My sister's beauty and elegance captured the attention of every eye there, and I was as good as invisible. The way it should be. I didn't become overwhelmed or overly self conscious about my appearance, afraid, or apprehensive. I felt peace, love, and joy for my sister. It could not have been a more perfect day. At the dinner reception, that little voice in my head definitely challenged me, and although I didn't eat a full plate, I did manage to eat a few bites. Some people watched me walk away after I excused myself to use the bathroom, but no-one got up to escort me. I think Melinda was about to follow me but Amy did have my back, like she said she would and stepped right between us blocking Melinda in and quickly striking up a conversation with her. Amy trusted me, and whether Melinda did or not, didn't matter to me anymore. One day in the future I hoped Melinda and I would get along on better terms, but today was not about us, and I had nothing to prove. Following dinner, Amy and I danced and laughed, and I also danced with my dad, Phillip, Rick, my mother, and Steffanni. At about ten o'clock Steffanni and Rick had their final dance and went around the room to say their goodbyes before catching their flight to their secret honeymoon destination. When they finally reached the door, everyone crowded down the stairs following them, waving, blowing bubbles, throwing rice, and Steffani threw her bouquet over her left shoulder. She looked back just in time to see it land perfectly in my crossed arms, and laughed hysterically blowing a wide kiss. Then moments later she was gone, and the remaining crowd had moved back inside to continue the party.

I said my goodbyes to everyone with promises to call far more often, and to let everyone know when I had visitor privileges so they could come to visit me.

"Well," Amy asked on the way back to Caitlynne's Place, "Anything you want to talk about before we get back?"

"No, but maybe we could take a small detour if you think that would be okay?"

"That depends. What did you have in mind?" She asked.

Half an hour later Amy pulled the car into a different church parking lot. It was a dark fall night, but the stars were brightly shining, and it was still warm from the days' sun. Still familiar with each bend and turn, I quickly found the path I had walked down not so long before, and made my way to Ameliah's resting place. I crouched down, and brushed some early fall leaves from the glossy black stone.

"Hey friend, you missed one heck of a party today. I can't stay long because Amy is waiting in the car for me and we have to get back to the house. I wanted to bring you this though, because I know they're you're favourite." I placed one lavender, thorn-less rose under her engraved name in the stone. "I miss you so much Ameliah. I'm doing okay, but things sure aren't the same in the house without you. I've been reading your journal you left me, and your prose is so reflective it really forces me to look deeper in myself at things. Some days are so much harder than others, but I'm going to do it. I know I have a long way to go, but I am going to get better. I'm getting stronger every day I think, little by little, and I am going to win this battle and continue living for both of us. I hope that wherever you are now my friend, you are happy and free. Nothing can hurt you now."

I stood up and started walking back to the car when all of a sudden out of the North sky, the brightest, most luminous light I had ever seen, streaked through the darkness; casting a brilliant glow over the grounds.

"Did you see that?" Amy called over to me excitedly.

"I sure did!" I shouted back smiling.

"That was so beautiful!"

It was beautiful indeed, and I also knew it was her. Ameliah had earned her wings. She had learned to love to fly.